"I cannot forbear a momentary tribute to Wentworth Higginson. Devoting himself heroically to his great work, absorbed in its duties, and bearing his oppressive responsibility as the leader of a regiment in which to a great extent are now involved the fortunes of a race, he adds another honorable name to the true chivalry of our time"

("Mr Pierce, on the Freedmen of Port Royal,"
Atlantic monthly for Sept. 1863)

OUT-DOOR PAPERS

BY

THOMAS WENTWORTH HIGGINSON

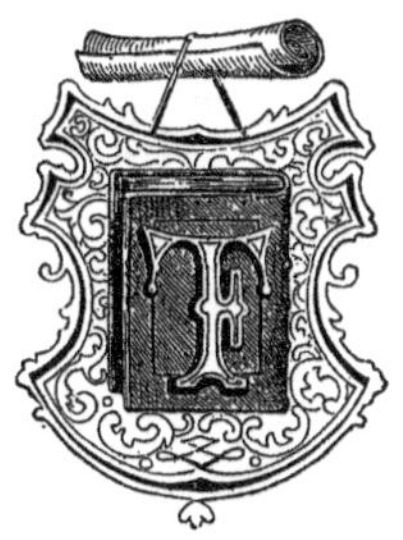

BOSTON
TICKNOR AND FIELDS
1863

UNIVERSITY PRESS:
WELCH, BIGELOW, AND COMPANY,
CAMBRIDGE.

Contents.

SAINTS, AND THEIR BODIES.

SAINTS, AND THEIR BODIES.

EVER since the time of that dyspeptic heathen, Plotinus, the saints have been "ashamed of their bodies." What is worse, they have usually had reason for the shame. Of the four famous Latin fathers, Jerome describes his own limbs as misshapen, his skin as squalid, his bones as scarcely holding together; while Gregory the Great speaks in his Epistles of his own large size, as contrasted with his weakness and infirmities. Three of the four Greek fathers — Chrysostom, Basil, and Gregory Nazianzen — ruined their health early, and were invalids for the remainder of their days. Three only of the whole eight were able-bodied men, — Ambrose, Augustine, and Athanasius; and the permanent influence of these three has been far greater, for good or for evil, than that of all the others put together.

Robust military saints there have doubtless been in the Roman Catholic Church: George, Michael, Sebastian, Eustace, Martin, Hubert the Hunter, and Christopher the Christian Hercules. But these have always held a very secondary place in canonization. Maurice and his whole Theban legion also were sainted together, to the number of six thousand six hundred and sixty-six; doubtless they were stalwart men, but there never yet has been a chapel erected to one of them. The mediæval type of sanctity was a strong soul in a weak body; and it could be intensified either by strengthening the one or by further debilitating the other. The glory lay in contrast, not in combination. Yet, to do them justice, they conceded a strong and stately beauty to their female saints, — Catherine, Agnes, Agatha, Barbara, Cecilia, and the rest. It was reserved for the modern Pre-Raphaelites to attempt the combination of a maximum of saintliness with a minimum of pulmonary and digestive capacity.

But, indeed, from that day to this, the saints by spiritual laws have usually been sinners against physical laws, and the artists have merely followed the examples they found. Vasari records, that Carotto's masterpiece of painting, "The Three Archangels," at Verona, was criticised because the limbs of the angels were too slender, and Carotto, true to his conventional standard, replied, "Then they will fly the better." Saints have been flying to heaven, for the same reason, ever since, — and have commonly flown young.

Indeed, the earlier some such saints cast off their bodies the better, they make so little use of them. Chittagutta, the Buddhist recluse, dwelt in a cave in Ceylon. His devout visitors one day remarked on the miraculous beauty of the legendary paintings, representing scenes from the life of Buddha, which adorned the walls. The holy man informed them that, during his sixty years' residence in the cave, he had been too much absorbed in meditation to notice the existence of the paintings, but he would take their word for it. And in this non-intercourse with the visible world there has been an apostolical succession, extending from Chittagutta down to the Andover divinity-student who refused to join his companions in their admiring gaze on that wonderful autumnal landscape which spreads itself before the Seminary Hill in October, but marched back into the library, ejaculating, "Lord, turn thou mine eyes from beholding vanity!"

It is to be reluctantly recorded, in fact, that the Protestant saints have not ordinarily had much to boast of, in physical stamina, as compared with the Roman Catholic. They have not got far beyond Plotinus. It is scarcely worth while to quote Calvin on this point, for he, as everybody knows, was an invalid for his whole lifetime. But it does seem hard that the jovial Luther, in the midst of his ale and skittles, should have deliberately censured Juvenal's *mens sana in corpore sano*, as a pagan maxim!

If Saint Luther fails us, where are the advocates of the body to look for comfort? Nothing this side of ancient Greece, we fear, will afford adequate examples of the union of saintly souls and strong bodies. Pythagoras the sage may or may not have been identical with Pythagoras the inventor of pugilism, and he was, at any rate, (in the loving words of Bentley,) "a lusty proper man, and built, as it were, to make a good boxer." Cleanthes, whose sublime "Prayer" is, doubtless, the highest strain left of early piety, was a boxer likewise. Plato was a famous wrestler, and Socrates was unequalled for his military endurance. Nor was one of these, like their puny follower Plotinus, too weak-sighted to revise his own manuscripts.

It would be tedious to analyze the causes of this modern deterioration of the saints. The fact is clear. There is in the community an impression that physical vigor and spiritual sanctity are incompatible. Recent ecclesiastical history records that a young Orthodox divine lost his parish by swimming the Merrimac River, and that another was compelled to ask a dismissal in consequence of vanquishing his most influential parishioner in a game of ten-pins; it seemed to the beaten party very unclerical. The writer further remembers a match, in a certain seaside bowling-alley, in which two brothers, young divines, took part. The sides being made up, with the exception of these two players, it was necessary to find places for them also. The head of one side accordingly picked his man, on the avowed presumption that the best preacher would naturally be the worst bowler. The athletic capacity, he thought, would be in inverse ratio to the sanctity. It is a satisfaction to add, that in this case his hopes were signally disappointed. But it shows which way the popular impression lies.

The poets have probably assisted in maintaining the delusion. How many cases of consumption Wordsworth must have accelerated by his assertion that "the good die first"! Happily he lived to disprove his own maxim. Professor Peirce has proved by statistics that the best scholars in our colleges survive the rest; virtue, like intellect, doubtless tends to longevity. The experience of the literary class shows that all excess is destructive, and that we need the harmonious action of all the faculties. Of the brilliant roll of the "young men of 1830," in Paris, — Balzac, Soulié, De Musset, De Bernard, Sue, and their compeers, — it is said that nearly every one has already perished, in the prime of life. What is the explanation? A stern one: opium, tobacco, wine, and licentiousness. "All died of softening of the brain or spinal marrow, or swelling of the heart." No doubt many of the noble and the pure were dying prematurely at the same time; but it proceeded from the same essential cause: physical laws disobeyed and bodies exhausted.

The evil is, that what in the debauchee is condemned, as suicide, is lauded in the devotee, as saintship. The *delirium tremens* of the drunkard conveys scarcely a sterner moral lesson than the second childishness of the pure and abstemious Southey.

But, happily, times change, and saints with them. Our moral conceptions are expanding to take in that "athletic virtue" of the Greeks, ἀρετὴ γυμναστική, which Dr. Arnold, by precept and practice, defended. The modern English "Broad Church" aims at breadth of shoulders, as well as of doctrines. Our American saintship, also, is beginning to have a body to it, a "Body of Divinity," indeed. Look at our three great popular preachers. The vigor of the paternal blacksmith still swings the sinewy arm of Beecher; Parker performed the labors, mental and physical, of four able-bodied men, until even his great strength yielded; and if ever dyspepsia attack the burly frame of Chapin, we fancy that dyspepsia will get the worst of it.

This is as it should be. One of the most potent causes of the ill-concealed alienation between the clergy and the people, in our community, is the supposed deficiency, on the part of the former, of a vigorous, manly life. There is a certain moral and physical *anhæmia*, this bloodlessness, which separates most of our saints, more effectually than a cloister, from the strong life of the age. What satirists upon religion are those parents who say of their pallid, puny, sedentary, lifeless, joyless little offspring, "He is born for a minister," while the ruddy, the brave, and the strong are as promptly assigned to a secular career! Never yet did an ill-starred young saint waste his Saturday afternoons in preaching sermons in the garret to his deluded little sisters and their dolls, without living to repent it in maturity. These precocious little sentimentalists wither away like blanched potato-plants in a cellar; and then comes some vigorous youth from his out-door work or play, and grasps the rudder of the age, as he grasped the oar, the bat, or the plough.

Everybody admires the physical training of military and naval schools. But these same persons never seem to imagine that the body is worth cultivating for any purpose, except to annihilate the bodies of others. Yet it needs more training to preserve life than to destroy it. The vocation of a literary man is far more perilous than that of a frontier dragoon. The latter dies at most but once, by an Indian bullet; the former dies daily, unless he be warned in time, and take occasional refuge in the saddle and the prairie with the dragoon. What battle-piece is so pathetic as Browning's "Grammarian's Funeral"? Do not waste your gymnastics on the West Point or Annapolis student, whose whole life will be one of active exercise, but bring them into the professional schools and the counting-rooms. Whatever may be the exceptional cases, the stern truth remains, that the great deeds of the world can be more easily done by illiterate men than by sickly ones. Wisely said Horace Mann, "All through the life of a pure-minded but feeble-bodied man, his path is lined with memory's gravestones, which mark the spots where noble enterprises perished, for lack of physical vigor to embody them in deeds." And yet more eloquently it has been said by a younger American thinker, Wasson, "Intellect in a weak body is like gold in a spent swimmer's pocket, — the richer he would be, under other circumstances, by so much the greater his danger now."

Of course, the mind has immense control over physical endurance, and every one knows that among soldiers, sailors, emigrants, and woodsmen, the leaders, though more delicately nurtured, will often endure hardship better than the followers, — "because," says Sir Philip Sidney, "they are supported by the great appetites of honor." But for all these triumphs of nervous power a reaction lies in store, as in the case of the superhuman efforts often made by delicate women. And besides, there is a point beyond which no mental heroism can ignore the body, — as, for instance, in sea-sickness and toothache. Can virtue arrest consumption, or self-devotion set free the agonized breath of asthma, or heroic energy defy paralysis? More formidable still are those subtle influences of disease, which cannot be resisted, because their source is unseen. Voltaire declared that the fate of a nation had often depended on the good or bad digestion of a prime-minister; and Motley holds that the gout of Charles V. changed the destinies of the world.

But part of the religious press still clings to the objection, that admiration of physical strength belonged to the barbarous ages of the world. So it certainly did, and so the race was kept alive through those ages. They had that one merit, at least; and so surely as an exclusively intellectual civilization ignored it, the arm of some robust barbarian prostrated that civilization at last. What Sismondi says of courage is pre-eminently true of that bodily vigor which it usually presupposes: it is by no means the first of virtues, but its loss is more fatal than that of all others. "Were it possible to unite the advantages of a perfect government with the cowardice of a whole people, those advantages would be utterly valueless, since they would be utterly without security."

Physical health is a necessary condition of all permanent success. To the American people it has a stupendous importance, because it is the only attribute of power in which they are losing ground. Guarantee us against physical degeneracy, and we can risk all other perils, — financial crises, Slavery, Romanism, Mormonism, Border Ruffians, and New York assassins; "domestic malice, foreign levy, nothing" can daunt us. Guarantee to Americans health, and Mrs. Stowe cannot frighten them with all the prophecies of Dred; but when her sister Catherine informs us that in all the vast female acquaintance of the Beecher family there are not a dozen healthy women, one is a little tempted to despair of the republic.

The one drawback to satisfaction in our Public-School System is the physical weakness which it reveals and helps to perpetuate. One seldom notices a ruddy face in the school-room, without tracing it back to a Transatlantic origin. The teacher of a large school in Canada went so far as to declare to me, that she could recognize the children born this side the line by their invariable appearance of ill-health joined with intellectual precocity, — stamina wanting, and the place supplied by equations. Look at a class of boys or girls in our Grammar Schools; a glance along the line of their backs affords a study of geometrical curves. You almost long to reverse the position of their heads, as Dante has those of the false prophets, and thus improve their figures; the rounded shoulders affording a vigorous chest, and the hollow chest an excellent back.

There are statistics to show that the average length of human life is increasing; and facts to indicate a development of size and strength with advancing civilization. Indeed, it is generally supposed that any physical deterioration is local, being peculiar to the United States. But the "Englishwoman's Journal" asserts that "it is allowed by all, that the appearance of the English peasant, in the present day, is very different to [from] what it was fifty years ago; the robust, healthy, hard-looking country-woman or girl is as rare now as the pale, delicate, nervous female of our times would have been a century ago." And the writer proceeds to give alarming illustrations, based upon the appearance of children in English schools, both in city and country.

We cannot speak for England, but certainly no one can visit Canada without being struck with the spectacle of a more athletic race of people than our own. One sees a large proportion of rosy female faces and noble manly figures. In the shop-windows, in winter weather, hang snow-shoes, "gentlemen's and ladies' sizes." The street-corners inform you that the members of the "Curling Club" are to meet to-day at "Dolly's," and the "Montreal Fox-hounds" at St. Lawrence Hall to-morrow. And next day comes off the annual steeple-chase, at the "Mile-End Course," ridden by gentlemen of the city with their own horses; a scene, by the way, whose exciting interest can scarcely be conceived by those accustomed only to "trials of speed" at agricultural exhibitions. Everything indicates out-door habits and athletic constitutions.

All this may be met by the alleged distinction between a good idle constitution and a good working constitution, — since the latter often belongs to persons who make no show of physical powers. But this only means that there are different temperaments and types of physical organization, while, within the limits of each, the distinction between a healthy and a diseased condition still holds; and it is that alone which is essential.

More specious is the claim of the Fourth-of-July orators, that, health or no health, it is the sallow Americans, and not the robust English, who are really leading the world. But this, again, is a question of temperaments. The Englishman concedes the greater intensity, but prefers a more solid and permanent power. He justly sets the noble masonry and vast canals of Montreal, against the Aladdin's palaces of Chicago. "I observe," admits the Englishman, "that an American can accomplish more, at a single effort, than any other man on earth; but I also observe that he exhausts himself in the achievement. Kane, a delicate invalid, astounds the world by his two Arctic winters, — and then dies in tropical Cuba." The solution is simple; nervous energy is grand, and so is muscular power; combine the two, and you move the world.

One may assume as admitted, therefore, the deficiency of physical health in America, and the need of a great amendment. But into the general question of cause and cure it is not here needful to enter. In view of the vast variety of special theories, and the inadequacy of any one, (or any dozen,) it is wiser to forbear. Perhaps the best diagnosis of the universal American disease is to be found in Andral's famous description of the cholera: "Anatomical characteristics, insufficient; — cause, mysterious; — nature, hypothetical; — symptoms, characteristic; — diagnosis, easy; — *treatment, very doubtful.*"

Every man must have his hobby, however, and it is a great deal to ride only one hobby at a time. For the present the writer disavows all minor ones. He forbears giving his pet arguments in defence of animal food, and in opposition to tobacco, coffee, and india-rubbers. He will not criticise the old-school physician whom he once knew, who boasted of not having performed a thorough ablution for twenty-five years; nor will he question the physiological orthodoxy of Miss Sedgwick's New England artist, who represented the Goddess of Health with a pair of flannel drawers on. Still less is it needful to debate, or to taste, Kennedy's Medical Discovery, or R. R. R., or the Cow Pepsin.

> "The wise for cure on *exercise* depend,"

saith Dryden, — and that is the argument now in question.

A great physician has said, "I know not which is most indispensable for the support of the frame, — food or exercise." But who, in this community, really takes exercise? Even the mechanic commonly confines himself to one set of muscles; the blacksmith acquires strength in his right arm, and the dancing-master in his left leg. But the professional or business man, what muscles has he at all? The tradition, that Phidippides ran from Athens to Sparta, one hundred and twenty miles, in two days, seems to us Americans as mythical as the Golden Fleece. Even to ride sixty miles in a day, to walk thirty, to run five, or to swim one, would cost most men among us a fit of illness, and many their lives. Let any man test his physical condition, either, if he likes work, by sawing his own cord of wood, or, if he prefers play, by an hour in the gymnasium or at cricket, and his enfeebled muscular apparatus will groan with rheumatism for a week. Or let him test the strength of his arms and chest by raising and lowering himself a few times upon a horizontal bar, or hanging by the arms to a rope, and he will probably agree with Galen in pronouncing it *robustum validumque laborem*. Yet so manifestly are these things within the reach of common constitutions, that a few weeks or months of judicious practice will renovate his whole system, and the most vigorous exercise will refresh him like a cold bath.

To a well-regulated frame, mere physical exertion, even for an uninteresting object, is a great enjoyment, which is, of course, qualified by the excitement of games and sports. To almost every man there is joy in the memory of these things; they are the happiest associations of his boyhood. It does not occur to him, that he also might be as happy as a child, if he lived more like one. What do most men know of the "wild joys of living," the daily zest and luxury of out-door existence, in which every healthy boy beside them revels? — skating, while the orange sky of sunset dies away over the delicate tracery of gray branches, and the throbbing feet pause in their tingling motion, and the frosty air is filled with the shrill sound of distant steel, the resounding of the ice, and the echoes up the hillsides? — sailing, beating up against a stiff breeze, with the waves thumping under the bow, as if a dozen sea-gods had laid their heads together to resist it? — climbing tall trees, where the higher foliage, closing around, cures the dizziness which began below, and one feels as if he had left a coward beneath and found a hero above? — the joyous hour of crowded life in football or cricket? — the gallant glories of riding, and the jubilee of swimming?

The charm which all have found in Tom Brown's "School Days at Rugby" lies simply in this healthy boy's-life which it exhibits, and in the recognition of physical culture, which is so novel to Americans. But efforts after the same thing begin to creep in among ourselves. A few Normal Schools have gymnasiums (rather neglected, however); the "Mystic Hall Female Seminary" advertises riding-horses; and we believe the new "Concord School" recognizes boating as an incidental; — but these are all exceptional cases, and far between. Faint and shadowy in early remembrance are certain ruined structures lingering Stonehenge-like on the Cambridge "Delta," — and mysterious pits adjoining, into which Freshmen were decoyed to stumble, and of which it is reported that vestiges still remain. Tradition spoke of Dr. Follen and German gymnastics; but the beneficent exotic was transplanted prematurely, and died. The only direct encouragement of athletic exercises which stands out in my memory of academic life was a certain inestimable shed on the "College Wharf," which was for a brief season the paradise of swimmers, and which, after having been deliberately arranged for their accommodation, was suddenly removed, the next season, to make room for coal-bins. Manly sports were not positively discouraged in those days, — but that was all.

Yet earlier reminiscences of the same beloved Cambridge suggest deeper gratitude. Thanks to thee, William Wells, — first pioneer, in New England, of true classical learning, — last wielder of the old English birch, — for the manly British sympathy which encouraged to activity the bodies, as well as the brains, of the numerous band of boys who played beneath the stately elms of that pleasant play-ground! Who among modern pedagogues can show such an example of vigorous pedestrianism in his youth as thou in thine age? and who now grants half-holidays, unasked, for no other reason than that the skating is good and the boys must use it while it lasts?

It is safe to cling still to the belief, that the Persian *curriculum* of studies — to ride, to shoot, and to speak the truth — is the better part of a boy's education. As the urchin is undoubtedly physically safer for having learned to turn a somerset and fire a gun, perilous though these feats appear to mothers, — so his soul is made healthier, larger, freer, stronger, by hours and days of manly exercise and copious draughts of open air, at whatever risk of idle habits and bad companions. Even if the balance is sometimes lost, and play prevails, what matter? It was a pupil of William Wells who wrote

> "The hours the idle school-boy squandered
> The man would die ere he 'd forget."

Only keep in a boy a pure and generous heart, and, whether he work or play, his time can scarcely be wasted. Which really has done most for the education of Boston, — Dixwell and Sherwin, or Sheridan and Braman?

Should it prove, however, that the cultivation of active exercises diminishes the proportion of time given by children to study, it is only an added advantage. Every year confirms the conviction, that our schools, public and private, systematically overtask the brains of the rising generation. We all complain that Young America grows to mental maturity too soon, and yet we all contribute our share to continue the evil. It is but a few weeks since the New York newspapers were shouting the praises of a girl's school, in that city, where the appointed hours of study amounted to nine and a quarter daily, and the hours of exercise to a bare unit. Almost all the Students' Manuals assume that American students need stimulus instead of restraint, and urge them to multiply the hours of study and diminish those of out-door amusements and of sleep, as if the great danger did not lie that way already. When will parents and teachers learn to regard mental precocity as a disaster to be shunned, instead of a glory to be coveted? One could count up a dozen young men who have graduated at Harvard College, during the last twenty years, with high honors, before the age of eighteen; and it is possible that nearly every one of them has lived to regret it. "Nature," says Tissot, in his Essay on the Health of Men of Letters, "is unable successfully to carry on two rapid processes at the same time. We attempt a prodigy, and the result is a fool." There was a child in Languedoc who at six years was of the size of a large man; of course, his mind was a vacuum. On the other hand, Jean Philippe Baratier was a learned man in his eighth year, and died of apparent old age at twenty. Both were monstrosities, and a healthy childhood would be equidistant from either.

One invaluable merit of out-door sports is to be found in this, that they afford the best cement for childish friendship. Their associations outlive all others. There is many a man, now perchance hard and worldly, whom one loves to pass in the street simply because in meeting him one meets spring flowers and autumn chestnuts, skates and cricket-balls, cherry-birds and pickerel. There is an indescribable fascination in the gradual transference of these childish companionships into maturer relations. It is pleasant to encounter in the contests of manhood those whom one first met at football, and to follow the profound thoughts of those who always dived deeper, even in the river, than one's own efforts could attain. There is a certain governor, of whom I personally can remember only that he found the Fresh Pond heronry, which I vainly sought; and in memory the august sheriff of a neighboring county still skates in victorious pursuit of me, (fit emblem of swift-footed justice!) on the black ice of the same lovely lake. My imagination crowns the Cambridge poet, and the Cambridge sculptor, not with their later laurels, but with the willows out of which they taught me to carve whistles, shriller than any trump of fame, in the happy days when Mount Auburn was Sweet Auburn still.

Luckily, boy-nature is too strong for theory. And truth demands the admission, that physical education is not so entirely neglected among us as the absence of popular games would indicate. It is very possible that this last fact proceeds partly from the greater freedom of field-sports in this country. There are few New England boys who do not become familiar with the rod or gun in childhood. Perhaps, in the mother country, the monopoly of land interferes with this, and that game laws, by a sort of spontaneous pun, tend to introduce games.

Again, the practice of match-playing is opposed to our national habits, both as a consumer of time, and as partaking too much of gambling. Still, it is done in the case of "firemen's musters," which are, we believe, a wholly indigenous institution. I have known a few cases where the young men of neighboring country parishes have challenged each other to games of base-ball, as is common in England; and there was a recent match at football between the boys of the Fall River and the New Bedford High Schools. And within a few years regattas and cricket-matches have become common events. Still, these public exhibitions are far from being a full exponent of the athletic habits of our people; and there is really more going on among us than this meagre "pentathlon" exhibits.

Again, a foreigner is apt to infer, from the more desultory and unsystematized character of our out-door amusements, that we are less addicted to them than we really are. But this belongs to the habit of our nation, impatient, to a fault, of precedents and conventionalisms. The English-born Frank Forrester complains of the total indifference of our sportsmen to correct phraseology. We should say, he urges, "for large flocks of wild fowl, — of swans, a *whiteness*, — of geese, a *gaggle*, — of brent, a *gang*, — of duck, a *team* or a *plump*, — of widgeon, a *trip*, — of snipes, a *wisp*, — of larks, an *exaltation*. The young of grouse are *cheepers*, — of quail, *squeakers*, — of wild duck, *flappers*." And yet, careless of these proprieties, Young America goes "gunning" to good purpose. So with all games. A college football-player reads with astonishment Tom Brown's description of the very complicated performance which passes under that name at Rugby. So cricket is simplified; it is hard to organize an American club into the conventional distribution of point and cover-point, long slip and short slip, but the players persist in winning the game by novel groupings and daring combinations. This constitutional independence has its good and evil results, in sports as elsewhere. It is this which has created the American breed of trotting horses, and which won the Cowes regatta by a mainsail as flat as a board.

But, so far as there is a deficiency in these respects among us, this generation must not shrink from the responsibility. It is unfair to charge it on the Puritans. They are not even answerable for Massachusetts; for there is no doubt that athletic exercises, of some sort, were far more generally practised in this community before the Revolution than at present. A state of almost constant Indian warfare then created an obvious demand for muscle and agility. At present there is no such immediate necessity. And it has been supposed that a race of shopkeepers, brokers, and lawyers could live without bodies. Now that the terrible records of dyspepsia and paralysis are disproving this, one may hope for a reaction in favor of bodily exercises. And when we once begin the competition, there seems no reason why any other nation should surpass us. The wide area of our country, and its variety of surface and shore, offer a corresponding range of physical training. Contrast our various aquatic opportunities, for instance. It is one thing to steer a pleasure-boat with a rudder, and another to steer a dory with an oar; one thing to paddle a birch-canoe, and another to paddle a ducking-float; in a Charles River club-boat, the post of honor is in the stern, — in a Penobscot *bateau*, in the bow; and each of these experiences educates a different set of muscles. Add to this the constitutional American receptiveness, which welcomes new pursuits without distinction of origin, — unites German gymnastics with English sports and sparring, and takes the red Indians for instructors in paddling and running. With these various aptitudes, we certainly ought to become a nation of athletes.

Thus it is that, in one way or another, American schoolboys obtain active exercise. The same is true, in a very limited degree, even of girls. They are occasionally, in our larger cities, sent to gymnasiums, — the more the better. Dancing-schools are better than nothing, though all the attendant circumstances are usually unfavorable. A fashionable young lady is estimated to traverse her three hundred miles a season on foot; and this needs training. But out-door exercise for girls is terribly restricted, first by their costume, and secondly by the social proprieties. All young female animals unquestionably require as much motion as their brothers, and naturally make as much noise; but what mother would not be shocked, in the case of her girl of twelve, by one tenth part the activity and uproar which are recognized as being the breath of life to her twin brother? Still, there is a change going on, which is tantamount to an admission that there is an evil to be remedied. Twenty years ago, if we mistake not, it was by no means considered "proper" for little girls to play with their hoops and balls on Boston Common; and swimming and skating have hardly been recognized as "lady-like" for half that period of time.

Still it is beyond question, that far more out-door exercise is habitually taken by the female population of almost all European countries than by our own. In the first place, the peasant women of all other countries (a class non-existent here) are trained to active labor from childhood; and what traveller has not seen, on foreign mountain-paths, long rows of maidens ascending and descending the difficult ways, bearing heavy burdens on their heads, and winning by the exercise such a superb symmetry and grace of figure as were a new wonder of the world to Cisatlantic eyes? Among the higher classes, physical exercises take the place of these things. Miss Beecher glowingly describes a Russian female seminary, in which nine hundred girls of the noblest families were being trained by Ling's system of calisthenics, and her informant declared that she never beheld such an array of girlish health and beauty. Englishwomen, again, have horsemanship and pedestrianism, in which their ordinary feats appear to our healthy women incredible. Thus, Mary Lamb writes to Miss Wordsworth, (both ladies being between fifty and sixty,) "You say you can walk fifteen miles with ease; that is exactly my stint, and more fatigues me"; and then speaks pityingly of a delicate lady who could accomplish only "four or five miles every third or fourth day, keeping very quiet between." How few

American ladies, in the fulness of their strength, (if female strength among us has any fulness,) can surpass this English invalid!

But even among American men, how few carry athletic habits into manhood! The great hindrance, no doubt, is absorption in business; and we observe that this winter's hard times and consequent leisure have given a great stimulus to out-door sports. But in most places there is the further obstacle, that a certain stigma of boyishness goes with them. So early does this begin, that the writer remembers, in his teens, to have been slightly reproached with juvenility, for still clinging to foot-ball, though a Senior Sophister. Juvenility! He only wishes he had the opportunity now. Mature men are, of course, intended to take not only as much, but far more active exercise than boys. Some physiologists go so far as to demand six hours of out-door life daily; and it is absurd to complain that we have not the healthy animal happiness of children, while we forswear their simple sources of pleasure.

Most of the exercise habitually taken by men of sedentary pursuits is in the form of walking. Its merits may be easily overrated. Walking is to real exercise what vegetable food is to animal; it satisfies the appetite, but the nourishment is not sufficiently concentrated to be invigorating. It takes a man out-doors, and it uses his muscles, and therefore of course it is good; but it is not the best kind of good. Walking, for walking's sake, becomes tedious. We must not ignore the *play-impulse* in human nature, which, according to Schiller, is the foundation of all Art. In female boarding-schools, teachers uniformly testify to the aversion of pupils to the prescribed walk. Give them a sled, or a pair of skates, or a row-boat, or put them on horseback, and they will protract the period of exercise till the complaint is transferred to the preceptor.

Gymnastic exercises have two disadvantages: one, in being commonly performed under cover (though this may sometimes prove an advantage as well); another, in requiring apparatus, and at first a teacher. Apart from these, perhaps no other form of exercise is so universally invigorating. A teacher is required, less for the sake of stimulus than of precaution. The tendency is almost always to dare too much; and there is also need of a daily moderation in commencing exercises; for the wise pupil will always prefer to supple his muscles by mild exercises and calisthenics, before proceeding to harsher performances on the bars and ladders. With this precaution, strains are easily avoided; even with this, the hand will sometimes blister and the body ache, but perseverance will cure the one and Russia Salve the other; and the invigorated life in every limb will give a perpetual charm to those seemingly aimless leaps and somersets. The feats once learned, a private gymnasium can easily be constructed, of the simplest apparatus, and so daily used; though nothing can wholly supply the stimulus afforded by a class in a public institution, with a competent teacher. In summer, the whole thing can partially be dispensed with; but it is hard for me to imagine how any person gets through the winter happily without a gymnasium.

For the favorite in-door exercise of dumb-bells we have little to say; they are not an enlivening performance, nor do they task a variety of muscles, — while they are apt to strain and fatigue them, if used with energy. Far better, for a solitary exercise, is the Indian club, a lineal descendant of that antique one in whose handle rare medicaments were fabled to be concealed. The modern one is simply a rounded club, weighing from four pounds upwards, according to the strength of the pupil; grasping a pair of these by the handles, he learns a variety of exercises, having always before him the feats of the marvellous Mr. Harrison, whose praise is in the "Spirit of the Times," and whose portrait adorns the back of Dr. Trall's Gymnastics. By the latest bulletins, that gentleman measured forty-two and a half inches round the chest, and employed clubs weighing no less than forty-seven pounds.

It may seem to our non-resistant friends to be going rather far, if we should indulge our saints in taking boxing lessons; yet it is not long since a New York clergyman saved his life in Broadway by the judicious administration of a "cross-counter" or a "flying crook," and we have not heard of his excommunication from the Church Militant. No doubt, a laudable aversion prevails, in this country, to the English practices of pugilism; yet it must be remembered that sparring is, by its very name, a "science of self-defence"; and if a gentleman wishes to know how to hold a rude antagonist at bay, in any emergency, and keep out of an undignified scuffle, the means are most easily afforded him by the art which Pythagoras founded. Apart from this, boxing exercises every muscle in the body, and gives a wonderful quickness to eye and hand. These same remarks apply, though in a minor degree, to fencing also.

Billiards is a graceful game, and affords, in some respects, admirable training, but is hardly to be classed among athletic exercises. Tenpins afford, perhaps, the most popular form of exercise among us, and have become almost a national game, and a good one, too, so far as it goes. The English game of bowls is less entertaining, and is, indeed, rather a sluggish sport, though it has the merit of being played in the open air. The severer British sports, as tennis and rackets, are scarcely more than names to us Americans, though both are to be practised in New York city.

Passing now to out-door exercises, (and no one should confine himself to in-door ones,) one must hold with the Thalesian school, and rank water first. Vishnu Sarma gives, in his apologues, the characteristics of the fit place for a wise man to live in, and enumerates among its necessities first "a Rajah" and then "a river." Democrats can dispense with the first, but not with the second. A square mile even of pond water is worth a year's schooling to any intelligent boy. A boat is a kingdom. I personally own one, — a mere flat-bottomed "float," with a centre-board. It has seen service, — it is eight years old, — has spent two winters under the ice, and been fished in by boys every day for as many summers. It grew at last so hopelessly leaky, that even the boys disdained it. It cost seven dollars originally, and I would not sell it to-day for seventeen. To own the poorest boat is better than hiring the best. It is a link to Nature; without a boat, one is so much the less a man.

Sailing is of course delicious; it is as good as flying to steer anything with wings of canvas, whether one stand by the wheel of a clipper-ship, or by the clumsy stern-oar of a "gundalow." But rowing has also its charms; and the Indian noiselessness of the paddle, beneath the fringing branches of the Assabeth or Artichoke, puts one into Fairyland at once, and Hiawatha's *cheemaun* becomes a possible possession. Rowing is peculiarly graceful and appropriate as a feminine exercise, and any able-bodied girl can learn to handle one light oar at the first lesson, and two at the second.

Swimming has also a birdlike charm of motion. The novel element, the free action, the abated drapery, give a sense of personal contact with Nature which nothing else so fully bestows. No later triumph of existence is so fascinating, perhaps, as that in which the boy first wins his panting way across the deep gulf that severs one green bank from another, (ten yards, perhaps,) and feels himself thenceforward lord of the watery world. The Athenian phrase for a man who knew nothing was, that he could "neither read nor swim." Yet there is a vast amount of this ignorance; the majority of sailors, it is said, cannot swim a stroke; and in a late lake disaster, many able-bodied men perished by drowning, in calm water, only half a mile from shore. At our watering-places it is rare to see a swimmer venture out more than a rod or two, though this proceeds partly from the fear of sharks, — as if sharks of the dangerous order were not far more afraid of the rocks than the swimmers of being eaten. But the fact of the timidity is unquestionable; and I was told by a certain clerical frequenter of a watering-place, himself an athlete, that he had never met but two companions who would swim boldly out with him, both being ministers, and one a distinguished Ex-President of Brown University. This fact must certainly be placed to the credit of the bodies of our saints.

But there is no space to descant on the details of all active exercises. Riding may be left to the eulogies of Mr. N. P. Willis, and cricket to Mr. Lillywhite's "Guide." It is pleasant, however, to see the rapid spread of clubs for the latter game, which a few years since was practised only by a few transplanted Englishmen and Scotchmen; and it is pleasant also to observe the twin growth of our indigenous American game of base-ball, whose briskness and unceasing activity are perhaps more congenial, after all, to our national character, than the comparative deliberation of cricket. Football, bating its roughness, is the most glorious of all sports to those whose animal life is sufficiently vigorous to enjoy it. Skating is just at present the fashion for ladies as well as gentlemen, and needs no apostle; it is destined to become a permanent institution.

A word, in passing, on the literature of athletic exercises; it is too scanty to detain us long. Five hundred books, it is estimated, have been written on the digestive organs, but it is hard to find half a dozen worth naming in connection with the muscular powers. The common Physiologies recommend exercise in general terms, but seldom venture on details; unhappily, they are written, for the most part, by men who have already lost their own health, and are therefore useful as warnings rather than examples. The first real book of gymnastics printed in this country, so far as we know, was the work of the veteran Salzmann, translated and published in Philadelphia, in 1802, and sometimes to be met with in libraries, — an odd, desultory book, with many good reasonings and suggestions, and quaint pictures of youths exercising in the old German costume. Like Dr. Follen's Cambridge gymnasium, it was probably transplanted too early, and produced no effect. Next came, in 1836, the book which is still, after twenty years, the standard, so far as it goes, — Walker's "Manly Exercises," — a thoroughly English book, and needing better adaptation to our habits, but full of manly vigor, and containing good and copious directions for skating, swimming, boating, and horsemanship. The only later general treatise worth naming is Dr. Trall's recently published "Family Gymnasium," — a good book, yet not good enough. On gymnastics proper it contains scarcely anything; and the essays on rowing, riding, and skating are so meagre, that they might almost as well have been omitted, though that on swimming is excellent. The main body of the book is devoted to the subject of calisthenics, and especially to Ling's system; all this is valuable for its novelty, although it is hard to imagine how a system so tediously elaborate can ever be made very useful for American pupils. Miss Beecher has an excellent essay on calisthenics, with very useful figures, at the end of her "Physiology." And on proper gymnastic exercises there is a little book so full and admirable, that it atones for the defects of all the others, — "Paul Preston's Gymnastics," — nominally a child's book, but so spirited and graphic, and entering so admirably into the whole extent of the subject, that it ought to be reprinted and find ten thousand readers.

These remarks have been purposely confined to those physical exercises which partake most of the character of sports. Field-sports alone have been omitted, as having been so often discussed by abler hands. Mechanical and horticultural labors lie out of the province of this essay. So do those of the artist and the man of science. The out-door study of natural history alone is a vast field, even yet very little entered upon. In how many American towns or villages are to be found *local collections* of natural objects, such as every large town in Europe affords, and without which the foundations of thorough knowledge cannot be laid? There are scarcely any. One finds innumerable fragmentary and aimless "Museums," — collections of South-Sea shells in inland villages, and of aboriginal remains in seaport towns, — mere curiosity-shops, which no man confers any real benefit by collecting; while the most ignorant person may be a true benefactor to science by forming a cabinet, however scanty, of the animal and vegetable productions of his own township. Professor Agassiz has often publicly lamented this waste of energy, and all may do their share to remedy the defect, while they invigorate their bodies by the exercise which the effort will give, and the joyous open-air life into which it will take them.

For, after all, the secret charm of all these sports and studies is simply this, — that they bring us into more familiar intercourse with Nature. They give us that *vitam sub divo* in which the Roman exulted, — those out-door days, which, say the Arabs, are not to be reckoned in the length of life. Nay, to a true lover of the open air, night beneath its curtain is as beautiful as day. The writer has personally camped out under a variety of auspices, — before a fire of pine logs in the forests of Maine, beside a blaze of faya-boughs on the steep side of a foreign volcano, and beside no fire at all (except a possible one of Sharp's rifles), in that domestic volcano, Kansas; and every such remembrance is worth many nights of in-door slumber. There is never a week in the year, nor an hour of day or night, which has not, in the open air, its own special interest. One need not say, with Reade's Australians, that the only use of a house is to sleep in the lee of it; but they might do worse. As for rain, it is chiefly formidable in-doors. Lord Bacon used to ride with uncovered head in a shower, and loved "to feel the spirit of the universe upon his brow"; and I once knew an enthusiastic hydropathic physician who loved to expose himself in thunder-storms at midnight, without a shred of earthly clothing between himself and the atmosphere. Some prudent persons may possibly regard this as being rather an extreme, while yet their own extreme of avoidance of every breath from heaven is really the more extravagantly unreasonable of the two.

It is easy for the sentimentalist to say, "But if the object is, after all, the enjoyment of Nature, why not go and enjoy her, without any collateral aim?" Because it is the universal experience of man, that, if we have a collateral aim, we enjoy her far more. He knows not the beauty of the universe, who has not learned the subtile mystery, that Nature loves to work on us by *indirections.* Astronomers say, that, when observing with the naked eye, you see a star less clearly by looking at it, than by looking at the next one. Margaret Fuller's fine saying touches the same point, — "Nature will not be stared at." Go out merely to enjoy her, and it seems a little tame, and you begin to suspect yourself of affectation. There are persons who, after years of abstinence from athletic sports or the pursuits of the naturalist or artist, have resumed them, simply in order to restore to the woods and the sunsets the zest of the old fascination. Go out under pretence of shooting on the marshes or botanizing in the forests; study entomology, that most fascinating, most neglected of all the branches of natural history; go to paint a red maple-leaf in autumn, or watch a pickerel-line in winter; meet Nature on the cricket-ground or at the regatta; swim with her, ride with her, run with her, and she gladly takes you back once more within the horizon of her magic, and your heart of manhood is born again into more than the fresh happiness of the boy.

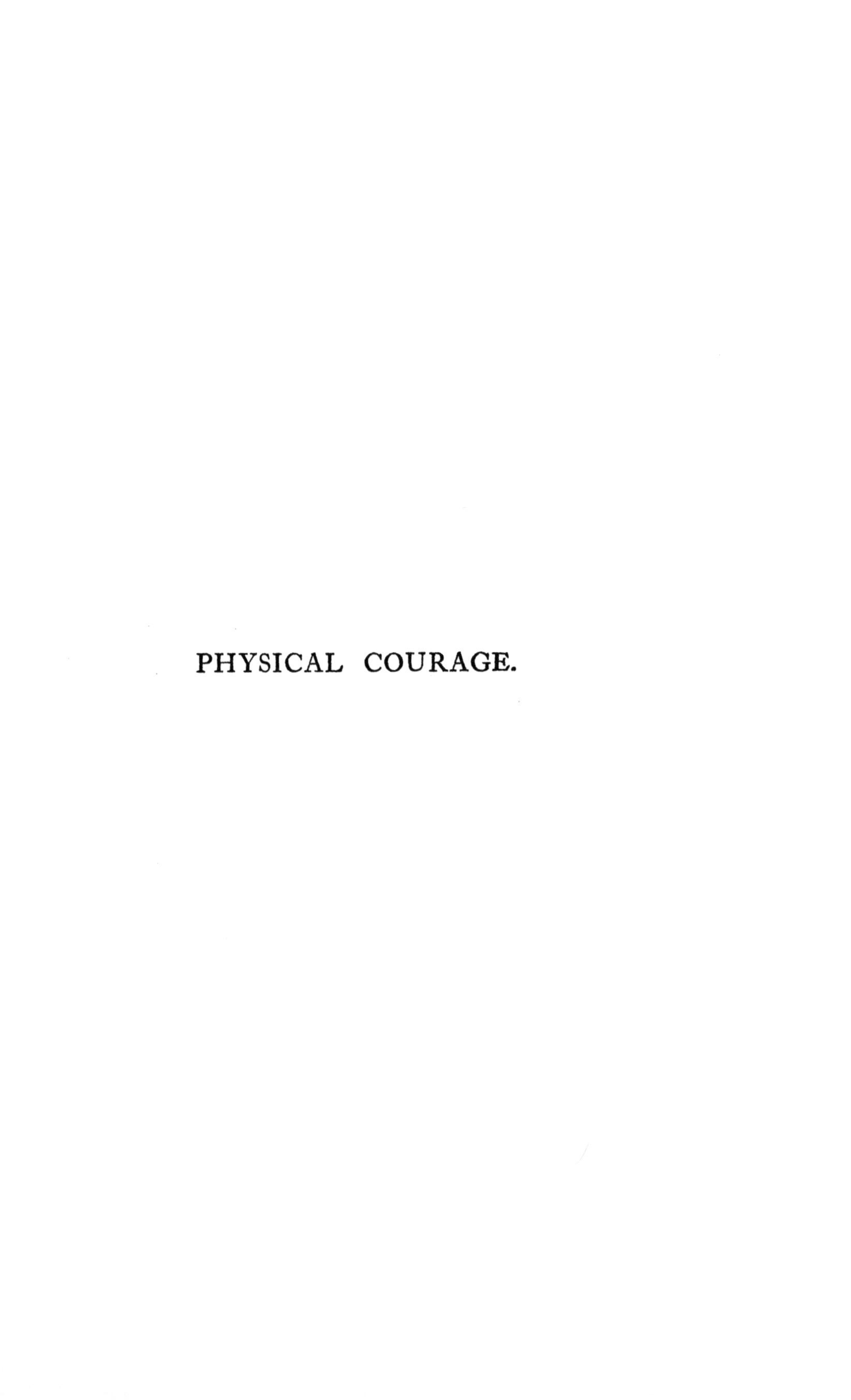

PHYSICAL COURAGE.

PHYSICAL COURAGE.

THE Romans had a military machine called a *balista*, a sort of vast crossbow, which discharged huge stones. It is said, that, when the first one was exhibited, an athlete exclaimed, "Farewell henceforth to all courage!" Montaigne relates, that the old knights, in his youth, were accustomed to deplore the introduction of fencing-schools, from a similar apprehension. Pacific King James predicted, but with rejoicing, the same result from iron armor. "It was an excellent thing," he said, — "one could get no harm in it, nor do any." And, similarly, there exists an opinion now, that the combined powers of gunpowder and peace are banishing physical courage, and the need of it, from the world.

Peace is good, but this result of it would be sad indeed. Life is sweet, but it would not be sweet enough without the occasional relish of peril and the luxury of daring deeds. Amid the changes of time, the monotony of events, and the injustice of mankind, there is always accessible to the poorest this one draught of enjoyment, — danger. "In boyhood," said the Norwegian enthusiast, Ole Bull, "I loved to be far out on the ocean in my little boat, for it was dangerous, and in danger one draws near to God." Perhaps every man sometimes feels this longing, has his moment of ardor, when he would fain leave politics and personalities, even endearments and successes, behind, and would exchange the best year of his life for one hour at Balaklava with the Six Hundred. It is the bounding of the Berserker blood in us, — the murmuring echo of the old death-song of Regnar Lodbrog, as he lay amid vipers in his dungeon: — "What is the fate of a brave man, but to fall amid the foremost? He who is never wounded has a weary lot."

This makes the fascination of war, which is in itself, of course, brutal and disgusting. Dr. Johnson says, truly, that the naval and military professions have the dignity of danger, since mankind reverence those who have overcome fear, which is so general a weakness. The error usually lies in exaggerating the difference, in this respect, between war and peace. Madame de Sévigné writes to her cousin, Bussy-Rabutin, after a campaign, "I cannot understand how one can expose himself a thousand times, as you have done, and not be killed a thousand times also." To which the Count answers, that she overrates the danger; a soldier may often make several campaigns without drawing a sword, and be in a battle without seeing an enemy, — as, for example, where one is in the second line, or rear guard, and the first line decides the contest. He finally quotes Turenne, and Maurice, Prince of Orange, to the same effect, that a military life is less perilous than civilians suppose.

It is, therefore, a foolish delusion to suppose, that, as the world grows more pacific, the demand for physical courage passes away. It is only that its applications become nobler. In barbarous ages, men fight against men and animals, and need, like Achilles, to be fed on the marrow of wild beasts. As time elapses, the savage animals are extirpated, the savage men are civilized; but Nature, acting through science, commerce, society, is still creating new exigencies of peril, and evoking new types of courage to meet them. Grace Darling at her oars, Kane in his open boat, Stephenson testing his safety-lamp in the terrible pit, — what were the trophies of Miltiades to these? And, indeed, setting aside these sublimities of purpose, and looking simply at the quantity and quality of peril, it is doubtful whether any tale of the sea-kings thrills the blood more worthily than the plain newspaper narrative of Captain Thomas Bailey, in the Newburyport schooner "Atlas," beating out of the Gut of Canso, in a gale of wind, with his crew of two men and a boy, up to their waists in the water.

It is easy to test the matter. Let any one, who believes that the day of daring is past, beg or buy a ride on the locomotive of the earliest express-train, some cold winter-morning. One wave of the conductor's hand, and the live engine springs snorting beneath you, as no Arab steed ever rushed over the desert. It is not like being bound to an arrow, for that motion would be smoother; it is not like being hurled upon an ocean crest, for that would be slower. You are rushing onward, and you are powerless; that is all. The frosty air gives such a brittle and slippery look to the two iron lines which lie between you and destruction, that you appreciate the Mohammedan fable of the Bridge Herat, thinner than a hair, sharper than a scimitar, which stretches over hell and leads to paradise. Nothing has passed over that perilous track for many hours; the cliffs may have fallen and buried it, the frail bridges may have sunk beneath it, or diabolical malice put obstructions on it, no matter how trivial, equally fatal to you; each curving embankment may hide unknown horrors, from which, though all others escape, you, on the engine, cannot; and still the surging locomotive bounds onward, beneath your mad career. You draw a long breath, as you dismount at last, a hundred miles away, as if you had been riding with Mazeppa or Brunechilde, and yet escaped alive. And there, by your side, stands the quiet, grimy engineer, turning already to his tobacco and his newspaper, and unconscious, while he reads of the charge at Balaklava, that his life is Balaklava every day.

Physical courage is not, therefore, a thing to be so easily set aside. Nor is it, as our reformers appear sometimes to assume, a mere corollary from moral courage, and, ultimately, to be merged in that. Moral courage is rare enough, no doubt, — probably the rarer quality of the two, as it is the nobler; but they are things diverse, and not necessarily united. There have been men, and still are such, leaders of their age in moral courage, and yet physically timid. This is not as it should be. God placed man at the head of the visible universe, and if he is to be thrown from his control, daunted by a bullet, or a wild horse, or a flash of lightning, or a lee shore, then man is dishonored, and the order of the universe deranged. No matter what the occasion of the terror is, a mouse or a martyrdom, fear dethrones us. "He that lives in fear of death," said Cæsar, "at every moment feels its tortures. I will die but once."

Having claimed thus much, it may still be readily admitted that we cannot yet estimate the precise effect upon physical courage of a state of permanent national peace, since indeed we are not quite within sight of that desirable consummation. Meanwhile, it is worth while to attempt some slight sketch and classification of the different types of this quality; — among which are to be enumerated the spontaneous courage of the blood, — the courage of habit or discipline, — magnetic or transmitted courage, — and the courage inspired by self-devotion or despair.

There is a certain innate fire of the blood, which does not dare perils for the sake of principle, nor grow indifferent to them from familiarity, nor confront them under support of a stronger will, — but loves them for their own sake, without reference to any ulterior object. There is no special merit in it, for it is a matter of temperament. Yet it often conceals itself under the finer names of self-devotion and high purpose, — as George Borrow convinced himself that he was actuated by evangelical zeal to spread the Bible in Spain, though one sees, through every line of his narrative, that it was chiefly the adventure which allured him, and that he would as willingly have distributed the Koran in London, had it been equally contraband. No surplices, no libraries, no counting-house desks, can eradicate this natural instinct. Achilles, disguised among the maidens, was detected by the wily Ulysses, because he chose arms, not jewels, from the travelling merchant's stores. In the most placid life, a man may pant for danger; and quiet, unobtrusive persons sometimes confess that they never step into a railroad-car without a sort of secret hope of a collision.

This is the courage of heroic races, as Highlanders, Circassians, Montenegrins, Afghans, and those Arabs among whom Urquhart finely said that peace could not be purchased by victory. Where destined to appear at all, it is likely to be developed in extreme youth, which explains such instances as the *gamins de Paris*, and that of Sir Cloudesley Shovel, who in boyhood conveyed a despatch during a naval engagement, swimming through double lines of fire. Indeed, among heroic races, young soldiers are preferable for daring; such, at least, is the testimony of the highest authorities, as Ney and Wellington. "I have found," said the Duke, "that raw troops, however inferior to the old ones in manœuvring, may be superior to them in downright hard fighting with the enemy. At Waterloo, the young ensigns and lieutenants, who had never before seen an enemy, rushed to meet death as if they were playing at cricket."

But though youth is good for an onset, it needs habit and discipline to give steadiness. A boy will risk his life where a veteran will be too circumspect to follow him; but to perform a difficult manœuvre in face of an enemy requires Sicinius with forty-five scars on his breast. "The very apprehension of a wound," said Seneca, "startles a man when he first bears arms; but an old soldier bleeds boldly, for he knows that a man may lose blood and yet win the day." Before the battle of Preston Pans, Mr. Ker of Graden, "an experienced officer," mounted on a gray pony, coolly reconnoitred all the difficult ground between the two armies, crossed it in several directions, deliberately alighted more than once to lead his horse through gaps made for that purpose in the stone walls, — under a constant shower of musket-balls. He finally returned unhurt to Charles Edward, and dissuaded him from crossing. Undoubtedly, any raw Highlander in the army would have incurred the same risk, with or without a sufficient object; but not one of them would have brought back so clear a report, — if, indeed, he had brought himself back.

The most common evidence of this frequent dependence of courage on habit is in the comparative timidity of brave men against novel dangers, — as of sailors on horseback, and mountaineers at sea. Nay, the same effect is sometimes produced merely by different forms of danger within the same sphere. Sea-captains often attach an exaggerated sense of peril to small boats; Condé confessed himself a coward in a street-fight; and William the Conqueror is said to have trembled exceedingly (*vehementer tremens*) during the disturbance which interrupted his coronation. It was probably from just the same cause, that Mrs. Inchbald, the most fearless of actresses, was once entirely overcome by timidity on assuming a character in a masquerade.

On a larger scale, the mere want of habitual exposure to danger will often cause a whole population to be charged with greater cowardice than really belongs to them. Thus, after the coronation of the Chevalier, in the Scottish insurrection of 1745, although the populace of Edinburgh crowded around him, kissing his very garments when he walked abroad, yet scarcely a man could be enlisted, in view of the certainty of an approaching battle with General Cope. And before this, when the Highlanders were marching on the city, out of a volunteer corps of four hundred raised to meet them, all but forty-five deserted before the gate was passed. Yet there is no reason to doubt that these frightened citizens, after having once stood fire, might have been as brave as the average. It was a saying in Kansas, that the New England men needed to be shot at once or twice, after which they became the bravest of the brave.

This habitual courage mingles itself, doubtless, with the third species, the magnetic, or transmitted. No mental philosopher has yet done justice to the wondrous power of leadership, the "art Napoleon." "There go thirty thousand men," shouted the Portuguese, as Wellington rode alone up the mountain-side, — and Wellington in turn used almost the same phrase in describing Napoleon to Rogers. The ancients stated it best in their proverb, that an army of stags led by a lion is more formidable than an army of lions led by a stag. It was for this reason that the Greeks used to send to Sparta, not for soldiers, but for a general. When Crillon, *l'homme sans peur*, defended Quillebœuf with a handful of men against the army of Marshal Villars, the latter represented to him, that it was madness to resist such superiority of numbers, to which the answer was simply, — "*Crillon est dedans, et Villars est dehors.*" The event proved that the hero inside was stronger than the army outside.

Every one knows that there is a certain magnetic power in courage, apart from all physical strength. In a family of lone women, there is usually some one whose presence is held to confer safety on the house: she may be a delicate invalid, but she is not afraid. The same quality explains the difference in the demeanor of different companies of men and women, in great emergencies of danger. Read one narrative of shipwreck, and human nature seems all sublime; read another, and, under circumstances equally desperate, it appears base, selfish, grovelling. The difference lies simply in the influence of a few leading spirits. Ordinarily, as is the captain, so are the officers, so are the passengers, so are the sailors. Bonaparte said, that at the beginning of almost every battle there was a moment when the bravest troops were liable to sudden panic; let the personal control of the general once lead them past that, and the field was half won.

The courage of self-devotion, lastly, is the faculty evoked by special exigencies, in persons who have before given no peculiar evidence of daring. It belongs especially to the race of martyrs and enthusiasts, whose personal terrors vanish in the greatness of the object, so that Joan of Arc, listening to the songs of the angels, does not feel the flames. This, indeed, is the accustomed form in which woman's courage proclaims itself at last, unsuspected until the crisis comes. This has given us the deeds of Flora Macdonald, Jane Lane, and the Countess of Derby; the rescue of Lord Nithisdale by his wife, and that planned for Montrose by Lady Margaret Durham; the heroism of Catherine Douglas, thrusting her arm within the stanchions of the doorway to protect James I. of Scotland, till his murderers shattered the frail barrier; and that sublimest narrative of woman's devotion, Gertrude Van der Wart at her husband's execution. It is possible that all these women may have been timid and shrinking before the hour of trial; and every emergency, in peace or war, brings out some such instances. At the close of the troubles of 1856 in Kansas, I chanced to be visiting a lady in Lawrence, who, in opening her work-basket, accidentally let fall a small pistol. She smiled and blushed, and presently acknowledged, that, when she had first pulled the trigger experimentally, six months before, she had shut her eyes and screamed, although there was only a percussion-cap to explode. Yet it afterwards appeared that she was one of the few women who remained in their houses, to protect them by their presence, when the town was entered by the Missourians, — and also one of the still smaller number who brought their rifles to aid their husbands in the redoubt, when two hundred were all that could be rallied against three thousand, in September of that eventful year. Thus easily is the transition effected!

This is the courage, also, of Africans, as manifested among ourselves, — the courage created by desperate emergencies. Suppled by long slavery, softened by mixture of blood, the black man seems to pass at one bound, as women do, from cowering pusillanimity to the topmost height of daring. The giddy laugh vanishes, the idle chatter is hushed, and the buffoon becomes a hero. Nothing in history surpasses the bravery of the Maroons of Surinam, as described by Stedman, or of those of Jamaica, as delineated by Dallas. Agents of the "Underground Railroad" report that the incidents which daily come to their knowledge are beyond all Greek, all Roman fame. These men and women, who have tested their courage in the lonely swamp against the alligator and the bloodhound, who have starved on prairies, hidden in holds, clung to locomotives, ridden hundreds of miles cramped in boxes, head downward, equally near to death if discovered or deserted, — and who have then, after enduring all this, gone voluntarily back to risk it over again, for the sake of wife or child, — what are we pale faces, that we should claim a rival capacity with theirs for heroic deeds? What matter, if none, below the throne of God, can now identify that nameless negro in the Tennessee iron-works, who, during the last insurrection, said "he knew all about the plot, but would die before he would tell? *He received seven hundred and fifty lashes, and died.*" Yet where, amid the mausoleums of the world, is there carved an epitaph like that?

The courage of blood, of habit, or of imitation, is not necessarily a very exalted thing. But the courage of self-devotion cannot be otherwise than noble, however wasted on fanaticism or delusion. It enters the domain of conscience. Yet, although the sublimest, it is not necessarily the most undaunted form of courage. It is vain to measure merit by martyrdom, without reference to the temperament, the occasion, and the aim. There is no passion in the mind of man so weak, said Lord Bacon, but it mates and masters the fear of death. Sinner, as well as saint, may be guillotined or lynched, and endure it well. A red Indian or a Chinese robber will dare the stake as composedly as an early Christian or an abolitionist. One of the bravest of all death-scenes was the execution of Simon, Lord Lovat, who was unquestionably one of the greatest scoundrels that ever burdened the earth. We must look deeper. The test of a man is not in the amount of his endurance, but in its motive; does he love the right, he may die in glory on a bed of down; is he false and base, these things thrust discord into his hymn of dying anguish, and no crown of thorns can sanctify his drooping head. Physical courage is, after all, but a secondary quality, and needs a sublime motive to make it thoroughly sublime.

Among all these different forms of courage it is almost equally true that it is the hardest of all qualities to predict or identify, in an individual case, before the actual trial. Many a man has been unable to discover, till the critical moment, whether he himself possessed it or not. It is often denied to the healthy and strong, and given to the weak. The pugilist may be a poltroon, and the bookworm a hero. I have seen the most purely ideal philosopher in this country face the dark muzzles of a dozen loaded revolvers with his usual serene composure. And on the other hand, I have known a black-bearded backwoodsman, whose mere voice and presence would quell any riot among the lumberers,—yet this man, nicknamed by his *employés* "the black devil," confessed himself to be in secret the most timid of lambs.

One reason of this difficulty of estimate lies in the fact, that courage and cowardice often complicate themselves with other qualities, and so show false colors. For instance, the presence or absence of modesty may disguise the genuine character. The unpretending are not always timid, nor always brave. The boaster is not always, but only commonly, a coward. Were it otherwise, how could we explain the existence of courage in Frenchmen or Indians? Barking dogs sometimes bite, as many a small boy, too trustful of the proverb, has found to his cost. "If that be a friend of yours," says Brantôme's brave Spanish Cavalier, "pray for his soul, for he has quarrelled with me." Indeed, the Gascons, whose name is identified with boasting, (gasconade,) were always among the bravest races in Europe.

Again, the mere quality of caution is often mistaken for cowardice, while heedlessness passes for daring. A late eminent American sculptor, a man of undoubted courage, is said to have always taken the rear car in a railroad train. Such a spirit of prudence, where well directed, is to be viewed with respect. We ought not to reverence the blind recklessness which sits on the safety-valve during a steamboat-race, but the cool composure which neither underrates a danger nor shrinks from it. The best encomium is that of Malcolm M'Leod upon Charles Edward, — "He was the most cautious man, not to be a coward, and the bravest man, not to be rash, that I ever saw"; or that of Charles VII. of France upon Pierre d'Aubusson, — "Never did I see united so much fire and so much wisdom."

Still again, men vary as to the form of danger which tests them most severely. The Irish are undoubtedly a brave nation, but their courage is apt to vanish in presence of sickness. They are not, however, alone in this, if we may judge from the newspaper statements, that, after the recent quarantine riots in New York, a small-pox patient lay all day untended in the Park, because no one dared to go near him. It is said of Dr. Johnson, that he was a hero against pain, but a coward against death. Probably the converse is quite as common. To a believer in immortality, death, even when premature, can scarcely be regarded as an unmitigated evil, but pain enforces its own recognition. One can hardly agree with the frightened recruit in the farce, who thinks "Victory or Death" a forbidding war-cry, but "Victory or Wooden Legs" a more appetizing alternative.

Besides these complications, there are those arising from the share which conscience has in the matter. "Thrice is he armed that hath his quarrel just," and the most resolute courage will sometimes quail in a bad cause, and even die in its armor, like Bois-Guilbert. It was generally admitted, on both sides, in Kansas, that the "Border Ruffians" seldom dared face an equal number; yet nobody asserted that these men were intrinsically deficient in daring; it was only conscience which made cowards of them all.

But it is, after all, the faculty of imagination which, more than all else, confuses the phenomena of courage and cowardice. A very imaginative child is almost sure to be reproached with timidity, while mere stolidity takes rank as courage. The bravest boy may sometimes be most afraid of the dark, or of ghosts, or of the great mysteries of storms and the sea. Even the mighty Charlemagne shuddered when the professed enchanter brought before him the vast forms of Dietrich and his Northern companions, on horseback. We once saw a party of boys tested by an alarm which appealed solely to the imagination. The only one among them who stood the test was the most cowardly of the group, who escaped the contagion through sheer lack of this faculty. Any imaginative person can occasionally test this on himself by sleeping in a large lonely house, or by bathing alone in some solitary place by the great ocean; there comes a thrill which is not born of terror, and the mere presence of a child breaks the spell, — though it would only enhance the actual danger, if danger there were.

This explains the effect of darkness on danger. "Let Ajax perish in the face of day." Who has not shuddered over the description of that Arkansas duel, fought by two naked combatants, with pistol and bowie-knife, in a dark room? One thrills to think of those first few moments of breathless, sightless, hopeless, hushed expectation, — then the confused encounter, the slippery floor, the invisible, ghastly terrors of that horrible chamber. Many a man would shrink from *that*, who would march coolly up to the cannon's mouth by daylight.

It is probably this mingling of imaginative excitement which makes the approach of peril often more terrible than its actual contact. "A true knight," said Sir Philip Sidney, "is fuller of gay bravery in the midst than at the beginning of danger." The boy Condé was reproached with trembling, in his first campaign. "My body trembles," said the hero, "with the actions my soul meditates." And it is said of Charles V., that he often trembled when arming for battle, but in the conflict was as cool as if it were impossible for an emperor to be killed. So Turenne was once asked by M. de Lamoignon, at the dinner-table of the latter, if his courage was never shaken at the commencement of a battle? "Yes," said Turenne, "I sometimes undergo great nervous excitement; but there are in the army a great multitude of subaltern officers and soldiers who experience none whatever."

To give to any form of courage an available or working value, it is essential that it have two qualities, promptness and persistency. What Napoleon called "two o'clock-in-the-morning courage" is rare. It requires great enthusiasm or great discipline to be proof against a surprise. It is said that Suwarrow, even in peace, always slept fully armed, boots and all. "When I was lazy," he said, "and wanted to enjoy a comfortable sleep, I usually took off one spur." In regard to persistency, history is full of instances of unexpected reverses and eleventh-hour triumphs. The battle of Marengo was considered hopeless, for the first half of the day, and a retreat was generally expected on the part of the French; when Desaix, consulted by Bonaparte, looked at his watch, and said, "The battle is completely lost, but it is only two o'clock, and we shall have time to gain another." He then made his famous and fatal cavalry-charge, and won the field. It was from a noble appreciation of this quality of persistency, that, when the battle of Cannæ was lost, and Hannibal was measuring by bushels the rings of the fallen Roman knights, the Senate of Rome voted thanks to the defeated general, Consul Terentius Varro, for not having despaired of the republic.

Thus armed at all points, incapable of being either surprised or exhausted, courage achieves results which seem miraculous. It is an element of inspiration, something superadded and incalculable, when all the other forces are exhausted. When we consider how really formidable becomes the humblest of quadrupeds, cat or rat, when it grows mad and desperate and throws all personal fear behind, it is clear that there must be a reserved power in human daring which defies computation and equalizes the most fearful odds. Take one man, mad with excitement or intoxication, place him with his back to the wall, a knife in his hand, and the fire of utter frenzy in his eyes, — and who, among the thousand bystanders, dares make the first attempt to disarm him? Desperate courage makes one a majority. Baron Trenck nearly escaped from the fortress of Glatz at noonday, snatching a sword from an officer, passing all the sentinels with a sudden rush, and almost effecting his retreat to the mountains; "which incident will prove," he says, "that adventurous and even rash daring will render the most improbable undertakings successful, and that desperate attempts may often make a general more fortunate and famous than the wisest and best-concerted plans."

It is this miraculous quality which helps to explain the extraordinary victories of history: as where the army of Lucullus at Tigranocerta slew one hundred thousand barbarians with the loss of only a hundred men, — or where Cortés conquered Mexico with six hundred foot and sixteen horse. The astounding narratives in the chivalry romances, where the historian risks his Palmerin or Amadis as readily against twenty giants as one, secure of bringing him safely through, — or the corresponding modern marvels of Alexandre Dumas, — seem scarcely exaggerations of actual events. A Portuguese, at the siege of Goa, inserted a burning match in a cask of gunpowder, then grasped it in his arms, and, crying to his companions, "Stand aside, I bear my own and many men's lives," threw it among the enemy, of whom a hundred were killed by the explosion, the bearer being left unhurt. John Haring, on a Flemish dike, held a thousand men at bay, saved his army, and finally escaped uninjured. And the motto of Bayard, *Vires agminis unus habet*, was given him after singly defending a bridge against two hundred Spaniards. Such men appear to bear charmed lives, and to be identical with the laws of Fate. "What a soldier, what a Roman, was thy father, my young bride! How could they who never saw him have discoursed so rightly upon virtue?"

From popular want of faith in these infinite resources of daring, it is a common thing for persons of eminent courage to be stigmatized as rash. This has been strikingly the case, for instance, in modern times, with the Marquis of Wellesley and Sir Charles Napier. When the Duke of Wellington was in the Peninsula in 1810, the City of London addressed the throne, protesting against the bestowal of "honorable distinctions upon a general who had thus far exhibited, with equal rashness and ostentation, nothing but an useless valor."

But if bravery is liable to exist in excess, on the one side, it is a comfort to think that it is capable of cultivation, where deficient. There may be a few persons born absolutely without the power of courage, as without the susceptibility to music, — but very few; and, no doubt, the elements of daring, like those of musical perception, can be developed in almost all. Once rouse the enthusiasm of the will, and courage can be systematically disciplined. Emerson's maxim gives the best regimen: "Always do what you are afraid to do." If your lot is laid amid scenes of peace, then carry the maxim into the arts of peace. Are you afraid to swim that river? then swim it. Are you afraid to leap that fence? then leap it. Do you shrink from the dizzy height of yonder magnificent pine? then climb it, and "throw down the top," as they do in the forests of Maine. Goethe cured himself of dizziness by ascending the lofty stagings of the Frankfort carpenters. Nothing is insignificant that is great enough to alarm you. If you cannot think of a grizzly bear without a shudder, then it is almost worth your while to travel to the Rocky Mountains in order to encounter the reality. It is said that Van Amburgh attributed all his power over animals to the similar rule given him by his mother in his boyhood, — "If anything frightens you, walk up and face it." Applying this maxim boldly, he soon satisfied himself that man possessed a natural power of control over all animals, if he dared to exercise it. He said that every animal divined by unerring instinct the existence of fear in his ruler, and a moment's indecision might cost one's life. On being asked, what he should do, if he found himself in the desert, face to face with a lion, he answered, "If I wished for certain death, I should turn and run away."

Physical courage may be educated; but it must be trained for its own sake. We say again, it must not be left to moral courage to include it, for the two faculties have different elements, — and what God has joined, human inconsistency may put asunder. The disjunction is easy to explain. Many men, when committed on the right side of any question, get credit for a "moral courage," which is, in their case, only an intense egotism, isolating them from all demand for human sympathy. In the best cause, they prefer to belong to a party conveniently small, and, on the slightest indications of popular approbation, begin to suspect themselves of compromise. The abstract martyrdom of unpopularity is therefore clear gain to them; but when it comes to the rack and the thumbscrew, the revolver and the bowie-knife, the same habitual egotism makes them cowards. These men are annoying in themselves, and still worse because they throw discredit on the noble and unselfish reformers with whom they are identified in position. But even among this higher class there are differences of temperament, and it costs one man an effort to face the brute argument of the slung-shot, while another's fortitude is not seriously tested till it comes to facing the newspaper editors.

These are but a few aspects of a rich and endless theme, depicted more by examples than analysis, according to the saying of Sidney, that Alexander received more bravery of mind by the example of Achilles than by hearing the definition of fortitude. If the illustrations have seemed to be drawn too profusely from the records of battles, it is to be remembered, that, even if war be not the best nurse of heroisms, it is their best historian. The chase, for instance, though perhaps as prolific in deeds of daring as the camp, has found few Cummings and Gerards for annalists, and the more trivial aim of the pursuit diminishes the permanence of its records. The sublime fortitude of hospitals, the bravery shown in infected cities, the fearlessness of firemen and of sailors, these belong to those times of peace which have as yet few historians. But the deep foundations and instincts of courage are the same wherever exhibited, and it matters little whence the illustrations come. Doubtless, for every great deed ever narrated, there were a hundred greater ones untold; and the noblest valor of the world may sleep unrecorded, like the heroes before Homer.

But there are things which, once written, the world does not willingly let die; embalmed in enthusiasm, borne down on the unconquerable instincts of childhood, they become imperishable and eternal. We need not travel to visit the graves of the heroes: they are become a part of the common air; their line is gone out to all generations. Shakespeares are but their servants; no change of time or degradation of circumstance can debar us from their lesson. The fascination which every one finds in the simplest narrative of daring is the sufficient testimony to its priceless and permanent worth. Human existence finds its range expanded, when Demosthenes describes Philip of Macedon, his enemy: "I saw this Philip, with whom we disputed for empire. I saw him, though covered with wounds, his eye struck out, his collar-bone broken, maimed in his hands, maimed in his feet, still resolutely rush into the midst of dangers, ready to deliver up to Fortune any part of his body she might require, provided he might live honorably and gloriously with the rest." Would it not be shameful, that war should leave us such memories as these, and peace bequeath us only money and repose? True, "peace hath her victories, no less renowned than war." No less! but they should be infinitely greater. *Esto miles pacificus,* "Be the soldier of peace," was the priestly benediction of mediæval knights; and the aspirations of humaner ages should lead us into heroisms which Plutarch never portrayed, and of which Bayard and Sidney only prophesied, but died without the sight.

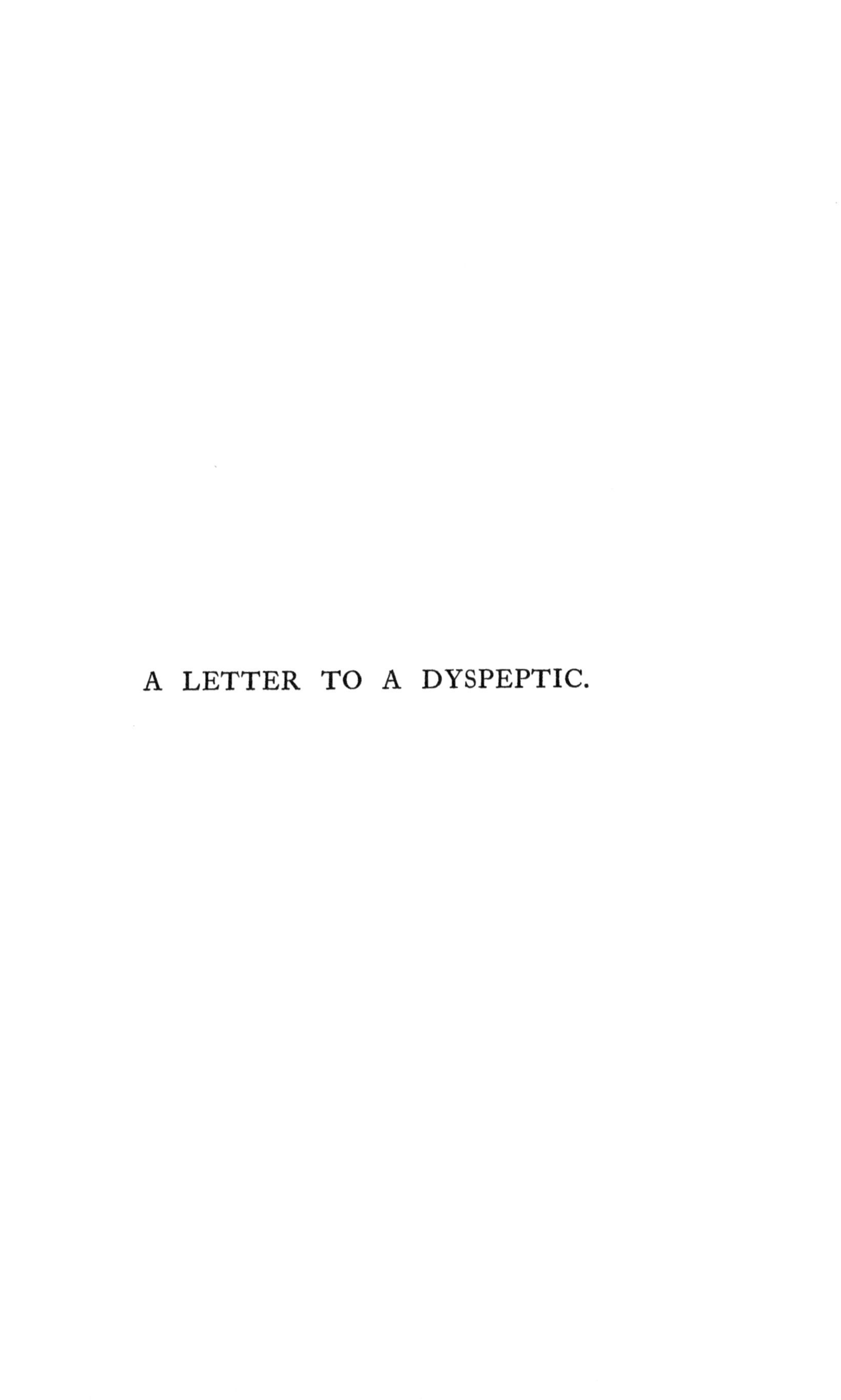

A LETTER TO A DYSPEPTIC.

A LETTER TO A DYSPEPTIC.

YES, my dear Dolorosus, I commiserate you. I regard your case, perhaps, with even sadder emotions than that excellent family-physician who has been sounding its depths these four years with a golden plummet, and has never yet touched bottom. From those generous confidences which, in common with most of your personal acquaintances, I daily share, I am satisfied that no description can do justice to your physical disintegration, unless it be the wreck of matter and the crush of worlds with which Mr. Addison winds up Cato's Soliloquy. So far as I can ascertain, there is not an organ of your internal structure which is in its right place, at present, or which could perform any particular service, if it were there. In the extensive library of medical almanacs and circulars which I find daily deposited by travelling agents at my front door, among all the agonizing vignettes of diseases which adorn their covers, and which Irish Bridget daily studies with inexperienced enjoyment in the front entry, there is no case which seems to afford a parallel to yours. I found it stated in one of these works, the other day, that there is iron enough in the blood of twenty-four men to make a broadsword; but I am satisfied that it would be impossible to extract enough from the veins of yourself and your whole family to construct a crochet-needle for your eldest daughter. And I am quite confident, that, if all the four hundred muscles of your present body were twisted together by a rope-maker, they would not furnish that patient young laborer with a needleful of thread.

You are undoubtedly, as you claim, a martyr to Dyspepsia; or if you prefer any other technical name for your disease or diseases, I will acquiesce in any, except, perhaps, the word "Neurology," which I must regard as foreign to etymological science, if not to medical. Your case, you think, is hard. I should think it would be. Yet I am impressed by it, I must admit, as was our adopted fellow-citizen by the contemplation of Niagara. He, you remember, when pressed to admire the eternal plunge of the falling water, could only inquire, with serene acquiescence in natural laws, "And what's to hinder?" I confess myself moved to similar reflections by your disease and its history. My dear Dolorosus, can you acquaint me with any reason, in the heavens above or on the earth beneath, why you should *not* have dyspepsia?

My thoughts involuntarily wander back to that golden period, five years ago, when I spent one night and day beneath your hospitable roof. I arrived, I remember, late in the evening. The bedroom to which you kindly conducted me, after a light but wholesome supper of doughnuts and cheese, was pleasing in respect to furniture, but questionable in regard to physiology. The house was not more than twenty years old, and the chamber must therefore have been aired within that distance of time, but not, I should have judged, more recently.

Perhaps its close, oppressive atmosphere could not have been analyzed into as many separate odors as Coleridge distinguished in Cologne, — but I could easily identify aromatic vinegar, damp straw, lemons, and dyed silk gowns. And, as each of the windows was carefully nailed down, there were no obvious means of obtaining fresh air, save that ventilator said to be used by an eminent lady in railway-cars, — the human elbow. The lower bed was of straw, the upper of feathers, whose extreme heat kept me awake for a portion of the night, and whose abundant fluffy exhalations suggested incipient asthma during another portion. On rising from these rather unrefreshing slumbers, I performed my morning ablutions with the aid of some three teacupsful of dusty water, — for the pitcher probably held that quantity, — availing myself, also, of something which hung over an elegant towel-horse, and which, though I at first took it for a child's handkerchief, proved on inspection to be "Chamber Towel, No. 1."

I remember, as I entered the breakfast-room, a vague steam as of frying sausages, which, creeping in from the neighboring kitchen, obscured in some degree the five white faces of your wife and children. The breakfast-table was amply covered, for you were always what is termed by judicious housewives "a good provider." I remember how the beefsteak (for the sausages were especially destined for your two youngest Dolorosi, who were just recovering from the measles, and needed something light and palatable) vanished in large rectangular masses within your throat, drawn downward in a maelstrom of coffee; — only that the original whirlpool is, I believe, now proved to have been imaginary; — "that cup was a fiction, but this is reality." The resources of the house also affòrded certain very hot biscuits or breadcakes, in a high state of saleratus; — indeed, it must have been from association with these, that certain yellow streaks in Mr. Ruskin's drawing of the rock, at the Athenæum, awakened in me such an immediate sense of indigestion; — also fried potatoes, baked beans, mince-pie, and pickles. The children partook of these dainties largely, but without undue waste of time. They lingered at table precisely eight minutes before setting out for school; though we, absorbed in conversation, remained at least ten; after which we instantly hastened to your counting-room, where you, without a moment's delay, absorbed yourself in your ledger, while I flirted languidly with the "Daily Advertiser."

You bent over your desk the whole morning, occasionally having anxious consultations with certain sickly men whom I supposed to be superannuated bookkeepers, in impoverished circumstances, and rather pallid from the want of nutritious food. One of them, dressed in rusty black, with a flabby white neckcloth, I took for an ex-clergyman; he was absorbed in the last number of the "Independent," though I observed, at length, that he was only studying the list of failures, a department to which, as it struck me, he himself peculiarly appertained. All of these, I afterwards ascertained from your office-boy, were eminent capitalists; something had gone wrong in the market, — not in the meat-market, as I should have supposed from their appearance, but in the money-market. I believe that there was some sudden fall in the price of indigo. I know you looked exceedingly blue as we walked home to dinner.

Dinner was ready the instant we opened the front door. I expected as much; I knew the pale, speechless woman who sat at the head of your table would make sure of punctuality, if she died for it. We took our seats without a word. Your eldest girl, Angelina, aged ten, one of those premature little grown women who have learned from the cradle that man is born to eat pastry and woman to make it, postponed her small repast till an indefinite future, and sat meekly ready to attend upon our wants. Nathaniel, a thin boy of eight, also partook but slightly, having impaired his appetite, his mother suspected, by a copious luncheon of cold baked beans and vinegar, on his return from school. The two youngest (twins) had relapsed to their couches soon after breakfast, in consequence of excess of sausage.

You were quite agreeable in conversation, I remember, after the first onset of appetite was checked. You gave me your whole theory of the indigo crisis, with minute details, statistical and geographical, of the financial condition and supposed present location of your principal absconding debtors. This served for what is called, at public dinners, the intellectual feast; while the carnal appetite was satisfied with fried pork, more and tougher beefsteak, strong coffee, cucumbers, potatoes, and a good deal of gravy. For dessert, (at which point Nathaniel regained his appetite,) we had mince-pie, apple-pie, and lemon-pie, the latter being a structure of a two-story description, an additional staging of crust being somehow inserted between upper and under. We lingered long at that noon meal, — fifteen minutes, at the very least; for you hospitably said that you did not have these little social festivals very often, — owing to frequent illness in the family, and other causes, — and must make the most of it.

I did not see much of you during that afternoon; it was a magnificent day, and I said, that, being a visitor, I would look about and see the new buildings. The truth was, I felt a sneaking desire to witness the match-game on the Common, between the Union Base-Ball Club, No. 1, of Ward Eleven, and the Excelsiors of Smithville. I remember that you looked a little dissatisfied, when I came into the counting-room, and rather shook your head over my narrative (perhaps too impassioned) of the events of the game. "Those young fellows," said you, "may not *all* be shiftless, dissipated characters *yet*, — but see what it comes to! They a'n't content with wasting their time, — they kill it, sir, actually kill it!" When I thought of the manly figures and handsome, eager faces of my friends of the "Union" and the "Excelsior," — the Excelsiors won by ten tallies, I should say, the return match to come off at Smithville the next month, — and then looked at the meagre form and wan countenance of their critic, I thought to myself, "Dolorosus, my boy, *you* are killing something besides Time, if you only knew it."

However, indigo had risen again, and your spirits also. As we walked home, you gave me a precise exhibit of your income and expenditures for the last five years, and a prospective sketch of the same for the next ten; winding up with an incidental delineation of the importance, to a man of business, of a good pew in some respectable place of worship. We found Mrs. D., as usual, ready at the table; we partook of pound-cake (or pound-and-a-half, I should say) and sundry hot cups of a very Cisatlantic beverage, called by the Chinese epithet of tea, — and went, immediately after, to a prayer-meeting. The church or chapel was much crowded, and there was a certain something in the atmosphere which seemed to disqualify my faculties from comprehending a single word that was spoken. It certainly was not that the ventilators were closed, for there were none. The minister occasionally requested that the windows might be let down a little, and the deacons invariably closed them again when he looked the other way. At intervals, females were carried out, in a motionless condition, — not, as it appeared, from conviction of sin, but from faintness. You sat, absorbed in thought, with your eyes closed, and seemed not to observe them. I remember that you were very much shocked when I suggested that the breath of an average sinner exhausted atmospheric air at the rate of a hogshead an hour, and asked you how much allowance the laws of the universe made for the lungs of church-members? I do not recall your precise words, but I remember that I finally found it expedient, as I was to leave for home in the early train, to spend that night at the neighboring hotel, where I indulged, on an excellent mattress, in a slumber so profound, that it seemed next morning as if I ought, as Dick Swiveller suggested to the single gentleman, to pay for a double-bedded room.

Well, that is all over now. You have given up business, from ill health, and exhibit a ripe old age, possibly a little over-ripe, at thirty-five. Your dreams of the forthcoming ten years have not been exactly fulfilled; you have not precisely retired on a competency, because the competency retired from you. Indeed, the suddenness with which your physician compelled you to close up your business left it closed rather imperfectly, so that most of the profits are found to have leaked out. You are economizing rather strictly, just now, in respect to everything but doctors' bills. The maternal Dolorosa is boarding somewhere in the country, where the children certainly will not have more indigestible food than they had at home, and may get less of it in quantity, — to say nothing of more air and exercise to aid digestion. They are not, however, in perfect condition. The twins are just getting up from scarlet fever; Nathaniel has been advised to leave school for a time; and something is thought to be the matter with Angelina's back. Meanwhile, you are haunting water-cures, experimenting on life-pills, holding private conferences with medical electricians, and thinking of a trip to the Bermudas.

You are learning, through all this, the sagest maxims of resignation, and trying to apply them. "Life is hard, but short," you say; "Providence is inscrutable; we must submit to its mysterious decrees." Would it not be better, my dear Dolorosus, to say instead, "Life is noble and immortal; God is good; we must obey his plain laws, or accept the beneficent penalties"? The rise and fall of health are no more accidental than the rise and fall of indigo; and it is the duty of those concerned in either commodity to keep their eyes open, and learn the business intelligently. Of the three proverbial *desiderata*, it is as easy to be healthy as to be wealthy, and much easier than to be wise, except so far as health and wisdom mean the same thing. After health, indeed, the other necessaries of life are very simple, and easily obtained; — with moderate desires, regular employment, a loving home, correct theology, the right politics, and a year's subscription to the "Atlantic Monthly," I have no doubt that life, in this planet, may be as happy as in any other of the solar system, not excepting Neptune and the fifty-five asteroids.

You are possibly aware, my dear Dolorosus, — for I remember that you were destined by your parents for the physician of your native seaside village, until you found a more congenial avocation in curing mackerel, — that the ancient medals represented the goddess Hygeia with a serpent three times as large as that carried by Æsculapius, to denote the superiority of hygiene to medicine, prevention to cure. To seek health as you are now seeking it, regarding every new physician as if he were Pandora, and carried hope at the bottom of his medicine-chest, is really rather unpromising. This perpetual self-inspection of yours, registering your pulse thrice a day, as if it were a thermometer and you an observer for the Smithsonian, — these long consultations with the other patients in the dreary parlor of the infirmary, the morning devoted to debates on the nervous system, the afternoon to meditations on the stomach, and the evening to soliloquies on the spine, — will do you no good. The more you know, under these circumstances, the worse it will be for you. You will become like Boerhaave's hypochondriacal student, who, after every lecture, believed himself to be the victim of the particular disease just expounded. We may even think too much about health, — and certainly too much about illness. I solemnly believe that the very best thing that could be done for you at this moment, you unfortunate individual, would be to buy you a saddle-horse and a revolver, and start you to-morrow for the Rocky Mountains, with distinct instructions to treat any man as a Border Ruffian who should venture to allude to the subject of disease in your presence.

But I cannot venture to hope that you will do anything so reasonable. The fascinations of your present life are too overwhelming; when an invalid once begins to enjoy the contemplation of his own woes, as you appear to do, it is all over with him. Besides, you urge, and perhaps justly, that your case has already gone too far, for so rough a tonic. What, then, can I do for you? Medicine I cannot offer; for even your respectable family-physician occasionally hints that you need something different from that. I suspect that all rational advice for you may be summed up in one prescription: Reverse instantly all the habits of your previous physical existence, and there may be some chance for you. But perhaps I had better enter more into detail.

Do not think that I am going to recur to the painful themes of doughnuts and diet. I fear my hints, already given, on those subjects, may wound the sensitive nature of Mrs. D., who suffers now such utter martyrdom from your condition that I cannot bring myself to heap further coals of fire on her head, even though the coals be taken from her own very ineffectual cooking-stove. Let me dwell rather on points where you have exclusive jurisdiction, and can live wisely or foolishly, at your pleasure.

It does not depend on you, perhaps, whether you shall eat bread or saleratus, meat or sole-leather; but it certainly does depend upon yourself whether you shall wash yourself daily. I do not wish to be personal, but I verily believe, O companion of my childhood! that, until you began to dabble in Hydropathy, you had not bestowed a sincere ablution upon your entire person since the epoch when, twenty years ago, we took our last plunge together, off Titcomb's wharf, in our native village. That in your well-furnished house there are no hydraulic privileges beyond pint water-pitchers, I know from anxious personal inspection. I know that you have spent an occasional week at the sea-shore during the summer, and that many people prefer to do up their cleanliness for the year during these excursions; indeed, you yourself have mentioned to me, at such times, with some enthusiasm, your daily sea-bath. But I have been privately assured, by the other boarders, that the bath in question always consisted of putting on a neat bathing-dress and sitting awhile on a rock among the sea-weed, like an insane merman, with the highest waves submerging only your knees, while the younger Dolorosi splashed and gambolled in safe shallows behind you. Even that is better than nothing, but — Soul of Mohammed! — is that called bathing? Verily, we are, as the Turks declare, a nation of "dirty Franks," if this be the accepted definition.

Can it be possible that you really hold with the once-celebrated Mr. Walker, "The Original," as he was deservedly called, who maintained that, by a correct diet, the system became self-purifying, through an active exhalation which repelled impurity, — so that, while walking on dusty roads, his feet, and even his stockings, remained free from dust? "By way of experiment, I did not wash my face for a week; nor did any one see, nor I feel, the difference." My deluded friend, it is a fatal error. Mr. Walker, the Original, may have been inwardly a saint and a sage, but it is impossible that his familiar society could have been desirable, even to fools or sinners. Rather recall, from your early explorations in Lemprière's Dictionary, how Medea renewed the youth of Pelias by simply cutting him to pieces and boiling him; whereon my Lord Bacon justly remarks, that "there may be some boiling required in the matter, but the cutting to pieces is not needful." If you find that the water-cure agrees with your constitution, I rejoice in it; I should think it would; but, I implore you, do not leave it all behind you when you leave the institution. When you return to your family, use your very first dollars for buying a sponge and a tin-hat, for each member of the household; and bring up the children to lead decent lives.

Then, again, consider the fact that our lungs were created to consume oxygen. I suppose that never in your life, Dolorosus, did those breathing organs of yours inhale more than one half the quantity of air that they were intended to take in, — to say nothing of its quality. Yet one would think, that, in the present high prices of food, you would make the most of the only thing you can put into your mouth gratis. Here is Nature constantly urging on us an unexceptionable atmosphere forty miles high, — for if a pressure of fourteen pounds to the square inch is not to be called urging, what is? — and yet we not only neglect, but resist the favor. Our children commonly learn to spell much better than they ever learn to breathe, because much more attention is paid to the former department of culture. Indeed, the materials are better provided; spelling-books are abundant; but we scarcely allow them time, in the intervals of school, to seek fresh air out of doors, and we sedulously exclude it from our houses and school-rooms. Is it not possible to impress upon your mind the changes which "modern improvements" are bringing upon us? In times past, if a gentleman finished the evening with a quiet cigar in his parlor, (a practice I deprecate, and introduce only for purposes of scientific illustration,) not a trace of it ever lingered to annoy his wife at the breakfast-table; showing that the draft up the open chimney had wholly disposed of it, the entire atmosphere of the room having been changed during the night. Now, on the other hand, every whiff lingers persistently beside the domestic altar, and betrays to the youngest child, next day, the parental weakness. For the sake of family example, Dolorosus, correct this state of things, and put in a ventilator. Our natures will not adapt themselves to this abstinence from fresh air, until Providence shall fit us up with new bodies, having no lungs in them. Did you ever hear of Dr. Lyne, the eccentric Irish physician? Dr. Lyne held that no house was wholesome, unless a dog could get in under every door and a bird fly out at every window. He even went so far as to build his house with the usual number of windows, and no glass in the sashes; he lived in that house for fifty years, reared a large family there, and no death ever occurred in it. He himself died away from home, of small-pox, at eighty; his son immediately glazed all the windows of the house, and several of the family died within the first year of the alteration. The story sounds apocryphal, I own, though I did not get it from Sir Jonah Barrington, but somewhere in the scarcely less amusing pages of Sir John Sinclair. I will not advise you, my unfortunate sufferer, to break every pane of glass in your domicile, though I have no doubt that Nathaniel and his boy-companions would enter with enthusiasm into the process; I am not fond of extremes; but you certainly might go so far as to take the nails out of my bedroom windows, and yet keep a good deal this side the Lyne.

I hardly dare go on to speak of exercise, lest I should share the reproach of that ancient rhetorician who, — as related by Plutarch, in his Aphorisms, — after delivering an oration in praise of Hercules, was startled by the satirical inquiry from his audience, whether any one had ever dispraised Hercules. As with Hercules, so with the physical activity he represents, — no one dispraises, if few practise it. Even the disagreement of doctors has brought out but little scepticism on this point. Cardan, it is true, in his treatise, "Plantæ cur Animalibus diuturniores," maintained that trees lived longer than men because they never stirred from their places. Exercise, he held, increases transpiration; transpiration shortens life; to live long, then, we need only remain perfectly still. Lord Bacon fell in with this fancy, and advised "oily unctions," to prevent perspiration. Maupertuis went farther, and proposed to keep the body covered with pitch for this purpose: conceive, Dolorosus, of spending threescore years and ten in a garment of tar, without even the ornament of feathers, sitting tranquilly in our chairs, waiting for longevity! In more recent times, I can remember only Dr. Darwin as an advocate of sedentary living. He attempted to show its advantages by the healthy longevity attained by quiet old ladies in country-towns. But this is questioned by his critic, Dr. Beddoes, who admits the longevity, but denies the healthiness; he maintains that the old ladies are taking some new medicine every day, — at least, if they have a physician who understands his business.

Now I will not maintain, with Frederick the Great, that all our systems of education are wrong, because they aim to make men students or clerks, whereas the mere shape of the body shows (so thought King Frederick) that we are primarily designed for postilions, and should spend most of our lives on horseback. But it is very certain that all the physical universe takes the side of health and activity, wooing us forth into Nature, imploring us hourly, and in unsuspected ways, to receive her blessed breath into body and soul, and share in her eternal youth. For this are summer and winter, seed-time and harvest, given; for this do violet and bloodroot come, and gentian and witch-hazel go; for this do changing sunsets make yon path between the pines a gateway into heaven; for this does day shut us down within the loneliness of its dome of light, and night, lifting it, make us free of the vast fellowship of stars; for this do pale meteors wander nightly, soft as wind-blown blossoms, down the air; for this do silent snows transform the winter woods to feathery things, that seem too light to linger, and yet too vast to take their flight; for this does all the fair creation answer to every dream or mood of man, so that we receive but what we give; — all is offered to us, to call us from our books and our trade, and summon us into Nature's health and joy. To study, with the artist, the least of her beauties, — to explore, with the man of science, the smallest of her wonders, — or even simply to wander among her exhaustless resources, like a child, needing no interest unborrowed from the eye, — this feeds body and brain and heart and soul together.

But I see that your attention is wandering a little, Dolorosus, and perhaps I ought not to be surprised. I think I hear you respond, impatiently, in general terms, that you are not "sentimental." I admit it; never within my memory did you err on that side. You also hint that you never *did* care much about weeds or bugs. The phrases are not scientific, but the opinion is intelligible. Perhaps my ardor has carried me too fast for my audience. While it would be a pleasure, no doubt, to see you transformed into an artist or a *savant*, yet that is scarcely to be expected, and, if attained, might not be quite enough. The studies of the naturalist, exclusively pursued, may tend to make a man too conscious and critical, — patronizing Nature, instead of enjoying her. He may even grow morbidly sensitive, like Buffon, who became so impressed with the delicacy and mystery of the human organization, that he was afraid to stoop even to pick up his own pen, when dropped, but called a servant to restore it. The artist, also, becomes often narrowed and petty, and regards the universe as a sort of factory, arranged to turn out good bits of color for him. Something is needed to make us more free and unconscious, in our out-door lives, than these too wise individuals; and that something is best to be found in athletic sports. It was a genuine impulse which led Sir Humphrey Davy to care more for fishing than even for chemistry, and made Byron prouder of his swimming than of "Childe Harold," and induced Sir Robert Walpole always to open his gamekeeper's letters first, and his diplomatic correspondence afterwards. Athletic sports are "boyish," are they? Then they are precisely what we want. We Americans certainly do not have much boyhood under the age of twenty, and we must take it afterwards or not at all.

Who can describe the unspeakable refreshment for an overworked brain, of laying aside all cares, and surrendering one's self to simple bodily activity? Laying them aside! I retract the expression; they slip off unnoticed. You cannot embark care in your wherry; there is no room for the odious freight. Care refuses to sit behind the horseman, despite the Latin sentence; you leave it among your garments when you plunge into the river, it rolls away from the rolling cricket-ball, the first whirl in the gymnasium disposes of it, and you are left free, as boys and birds are free. If athletic amusements did nothing for the body, they would still be medicine for the soul. Nay, it is Plato who says that exercise will almost cure a guilty conscience, — and can we be indifferent to this, my fellow-sinner?

Why will you persist in urging that you "cannot

afford" these indulgences, as you call them? They are not indulgences, — they are necessaries. Charge them, in your private account-book, under the heads of food and clothing, and as a substitute for your present enormous items under the head of medicine. O mistaken economist! can you afford the cessation of labor and the ceaseless drugging and douching of your last few years? Did not all your large experience in the retail business teach you the comparative value of the ounce of prevention and the pound of cure? Are not fresh air and cold water to be had cheap? and is not good bread less costly than cake and pies? Is not the gymnasium a more economical institution than the hospital? and is not a pair of skates a good investment, if it aids you to elude the grasp of the apothecary? Is the cow Pepsin, on the whole, a more frugal hobby to ride than a good saddle-horse? Besides, if you insist upon pecuniary economy, do begin by economizing on the exercise which you pay others for taking in your stead, — on the corn and pears which you buy in the market, instead of removing to a suburban house and raising them yourself, — and in the reluctant silver you pay the Irishman who splits your wood. Or if, suddenly reversing your line of argument, you plead that this would impoverish the Irishman, you can at least treat him as you do the organ-grinder, and pay him an extra fee to go on to your next neighbor.

Dolorosus, there is something very noble, if you could but discover it, in a perfect human body. In spite of all our bemoaning, the physical structure of man displays its due power and beauty when we consent to give it a fair chance. On the cheek of every healthy child that plays in the street, though clouded by all the dirt that ever incrusted a young O'Brien or M'Cafferty, there is a glory of color such as no artist ever painted. I can take you to-morrow into a circus or a gymnasium, and show you limbs and attitudes which are worth more study than the Apollo or the Antinoüs, because they are life, not marble. How noble were Horatio Greenough's meditations, in presence of the despised circus-rider! "I worship, when I see this brittle form borne at full speed on the back of a fiery horse, yet dancing as on the quiet ground, and smiling in conscious safety."

I admit that this view, like every other, may be carried to excess. We can hardly expect to correct our past neglect of bodily training, without falling into reactions and extremes in the process. There is our friend Jones, for instance, "the Englishman," as the boys on the Common call him, from his cheery portliness of aspect. He is the man who insisted on keeping the telegraph-office open until 2 A. M., to hear whether Morrissey or the Benicia Boy won the prize-fight. I cannot say much for his personal conformity to his own theories at present, for he is growing rather too stout; but he likes vicarious exercise, and is doing something for the next generation, even if he does make the club laugh, sometimes, by advancing theories of training which the lower circumference of his own waistcoat does not seem to justify. But Charley, his eldest, can ride, shoot, and speak the truth, like an ancient Persian; he is the best boxer in college, and is now known to have gone to Canada *incog.*, during the vacation, under the immediate supervision of Morris, the teacher of sparring, to see that same fight. It is true that the youth blushes, now, whenever that trip is alluded to; and when he was cross-questioned by his pet sister Kate, (Kate Coventry she delights to be called,) as to whether it was n't "splendid," he hastily told her that she did n't know what she was talking about, (which was undoubtedly true,) — and that he wished he did n't, either. The truth is, that Charley, with his honest, boyish face, must have been singularly out of place among that brutal circle; and there is little doubt that he retired from the company before the set-to was fairly begun, and that respectable old Morris went with him. But, at any rate, they are a noble-looking family, and well brought up. Charley, with all his pugilism, stands fair for a part at Commencement, they say; and if you could have seen little Kate teaching her big cousin to skate backwards, at Jamaica Pond, last February, it would have reminded you of the pretty scene of the little cadet attitudinizing before the great Formes, in "Figaro." The whole family incline in the same direction; even Laura, the elder sister, who is attending a course of lectures on Hygiene, and just at present sits motionless for half an hour before every meal for her stomach's sake, and again a whole hour afterwards for her often (imaginary) infirmities, — even Laura is a perfect Hebe in health and bloom, and saved herself and her little sister when the boat upset, last summer, at Dove Harbor, — while the two young men who were with them had much ado to secure their own elegant persons, without rendering much aid to the girls. And when I think, Dolorosus, of this splendid animal vigor of the race of Jones, and then call to mind the melancholy countenances of your forlorn little offspring, I really think that it would, on the whole, be unsafe to trust you with that revolver; you might be tempted to damage yourself or somebody else with it, before departing for the Rocky Mountains.

Do not think me heartless for what I say, or assume

that, because I happen to be healthy myself, I have no mercy for ill-health in others. There are invalids who are objects of sympathy indeed, guiltless heirs of ancestral disease, or victims of parental folly or sin, — those whose lives are early blighted by maladies that seem as causeless as they are cureless, — or those with whom the world has dealt so cruelly that all their delicate nature is like sweet bells jangled, — or those whose powers of life are all exhausted by unnoticed labors and unseen cares, — or those prematurely old with duties and dangers, heroes of thought and action, whose very names evoke the passion and the pride of a hundred thousand hearts. There is a tottering feebleness of old age, also, nobler than any prime of strength; we all know aged men who are floating on, in stately serenity, towards their last harbor, like Turner's Old Téméraire, with quiet tides around them, and the blessed sunset bathing in loveliness all their dying day. Let human love do its gracious work upon all these; let angelic hands of women wait upon their lightest needs, and every voice of salutation be tuned to such a sweetness as if it whispered beside a dying mother's bed.

But you, Dolorosus, — you, to whom God gave youth and health, and who might have kept them, the one long and the other perchance always, but who never loved them, nor reverenced them, nor cherished them, only coined them into money till they were all gone, and even the ill-gotten treasure fell from your debilitated hands, — you, who shunned the sunshine as if it were sin, and called all innocent recreation time wasted, — you, who stayed under ground in your gold-mine, like the sightless fishes of the Mammoth Cave, till you were as blind and unjoyous as they, — what plea have you to make, what shelter to claim, except that charity which suffereth long and is kind? We will strive not to withhold it; while there is life, there is hope. At forty, it is said, every man is a fool or a physician. We will wait and see which vocation you select as your own, for the broken remnant of your days.

THE

MURDER OF THE INNOCENTS.

A SECOND EPISTLE TO DOLOROSUS.

THE MURDER OF THE INNOCENTS.

SO you are already mending, my dear fellow? Can it be that my modest epistle has done so much service? Are you like those invalids in Central Africa, who, when the medicine itself is not accessible, straightway swallow the written prescription as a substitute, inwardly digest it, and recover? No, — I think you have tested the actual *materia medica* recommended. I hear of you from all directions, walking up hills in the mornings and down hills in the afternoons, skimming round in wherries like a rather unsteady water-spider, blistering your hands upon gymnastic bars, receiving severe contusions on your nose from cricket-balls, shaking up and down on hard trotting-horses, and making the most startling innovations in respect to eating, sleeping, and bathing. Like all our countrymen, you are plunging from one extreme to the other. Undoubtedly, you will soon make yourself sick again; but your present extreme is the safer of the two. Time works many miracles; it has made Louis Napoleon espouse the cause of liberty, and it may yet make you reasonable.

After all, that advice of mine, which is thought to have benefited you so greatly, was simply that which Dr. Abernethy used to give his patients: "Don't come to me,

—go buy a skipping-rope." If you can only guard against excesses, and keep the skipping-rope in operation, there are yet hopes for you. Only remember that it is equally important to preserve health as to attain it, and it needs much the same regimen. Do not be like that Lord Russell in Spence's Anecdotes, who only went hunting for the sake of an appetite, and who, the moment he felt any sensation of vitality in the epigastrium, used to turn short round, exclaiming, "I have found it!" and ride home from the finest chase. It was the same Lord Russell, by the way, who, when he met a beggar and was implored to give him something, because he was almost famished with hunger, called him a happy dog, and envied him too much to relieve him. From some recent remarks of your boarding-house hostess, my friend, I am led to suppose that you are now almost as well off, in point of appetite, as if you were a beggar; and I wish to keep you so.

How much the spirits rise with health! A family of children is a very different sight to a healthy man and to a dyspeptic. What pleasure you now take in yours! You are going to live more in their manner and for their sakes, henceforward, you tell me. You are to enter upon business again, but in a more moderate way; you are to live in a pleasant little suburban cottage, with fresh air, a horse-railroad, and good schools. For I am not surprised to find that your interest in your offspring, like that of most American parents, culminates in the school-room. This important matter you have neglected long enough, you think, while you were foolishly absorbed in making money for them. Now they shall have money enough, to be sure, but wisdom in superabundance. Angelina shall walk in silk attire, and knowledge have to spare.

To which school shall you send her? you ask me, with something of the old careworn expression, pulling six different prospectuses from your pocket. Put them away, Dolorosus; I know the needs of Angelina, and I can answer instantly. Send the girl, for the present at least, to that school whose daily hours of session are the shortest, and whose recess-times and vacations are of the most formidable length.

No, anxious parent, I am not joking. I am more anxious for your children than you are. On the faith of an ex-teacher and ex-school-committee-man, — for what respectable middle-aged American man but has passed through both these spheres of uncomfortable usefulness? — I am terribly in earnest. Upon this implied thesis, — that the merit of an American school, at least so far as Angelina is concerned, is in inverse ratio to the time given to study, — I will lay down incontrovertible reasonings.

Sir Walter Scott, according to Carlyle, was the only perfectly healthy literary man who ever lived, — in fact, the one suitable text, he says, for a sermon on health. You may wonder, Dolorosus, what Sir Walter Scott has to do with Angelina, except to supply her with novel-reading, and with passages for impassioned recitation, at the twilight hour, from "The Lady of the Lake." But that same Scott has left one remark on record which may yet save the lives and reasons of greater men than himself, more gifted women (if that were possible) than Angelina, if we can only accept it with the deference to which that same healthiness of his entitles it. He gave it as his deliberate opinion, in conversation with Basil Hall, that five and a half hours form the limit of healthful mental labor for a mature person. "This I reckon very good work for a man," he said, — adding, "I can very seldom reach six hours a day; and I reckon that what is written after five or six hours' hard mental labor is not good for much." This he said in the fulness of his magnificent strength, and when he was producing, with astounding rapidity, those pages of delight over which every new generation still hangs enchanted.

He did not mean, of course, that this was the maximum of possible mental labor, but only of wise and desirable labor. In later life, driven by terrible pecuniary anxieties, he himself worked more than this. Southey, his contemporary, worked far harder, — writing, in 1814, "I cannot get through more than at present, unless I give up sleep, or the little exercise I take (walking a mile and back, after breakfast); and, that hour excepted, and my meals, (barely the meals, for I remain not one minute after them,) the pen or the book is always in my hand." Our own time and country afford a yet more astonishing instance. Theodore Parker, to my certain knowledge, has often spent in his study from twelve to seventeen hours daily, for weeks together. But the result in all these cases has sadly proved the supremacy of the laws which were defied; and the nobler the victim, the more tremendous the warning retribution.

Let us return, then, from the practice of Scott's ruined days to the principles of his sound ones. Supposing his estimate to be correct, and five and a half hours to be a reasonable limit for the day's work of a mature intellect, it is evident that even this must be altogether too much for an immature one. "To suppose the youthful brain," says the recent admirable report, by Dr. Ray, of the Providence Insane Hospital, "to be capable of an amount of work which is considered an ample allowance to an adult brain, is simply absurd, and the attempt to carry this fully into effect must necessarily be dangerous to the health and efficacy of the organ." It would be wrong, therefore, to deduct less than a half-hour from Scott's estimate, for even the oldest pupils in our highest schools; leaving five hours as the limit of real mental effort for them, and reducing this, for all younger pupils, very much farther.

It is vain to suggest, at this point, that the application of Scott's estimate is not fair, because the mental labor of our schools is different in quality from his, and therefore less exhausting. It differs only in being more exhausting. To the robust and affluent mind of the novelist, composition was not, of itself, exceedingly fatiguing; we know this from his own testimony; he was able, moreover, to select his own subject, keep his own hours, and arrange all his own conditions of labor. And on the other hand, when we consider what energy and genius have for years been brought to bear upon the perfecting of our educational methods, — how thoroughly our best schools are now graded and systematized, until each day's lessons become a Procrustes-bed to which all must fit themselves, — how stimulating the apparatus of prizes and applauses, how crushing the penalties of reproof and degradation, — when we reflect, that it is the ideal of every school to concentrate the whole faculties of every scholar upon each lesson and each recitation from beginning to end, and that anything short of this is considered partial failure, — it is not exaggeration to say, that the daily tension of brain demanded of children in our best schools is altogether severer than that upon which Scott based his estimate. But Scott is not the only authority in the case; let us ask the physiologists.

So said Horace Mann, before us, in the days when the Massachusetts school system was in process of formation. *He* asked the physiologists, in 1840, and in his next Report printed the answers of three of the most eminent. The late Dr. Woodward, of Worcester, promptly said, that children under eight should never be confined more than one hour at a time, nor more than four hours a day; and that, if any child showed alarming symptoms of precocity, it should be taken from school altogether. Dr. James Jackson, of Boston, allowed the children four hours' schooling in winter and five in summer, but only one hour at a time, and heartily expressed his "detestation of the practice of giving young children lessons to learn at home." Dr. S. G. Howe, reasoning elaborately on the whole subject, said, that children under eight should not be confined more than half an hour at a time, — "by following which rule, with long recesses, they can study four hours daily"; children between eight and fourteen should not be confined more than three quarters of an hour at a time, having the last quarter of each hour for exercise in the playground; — and he allowed six hours of school in winter, or seven in summer, solely on condition of this deduction of twenty-five per cent for recesses.

Indeed, the one thing about which doctors do *not* disagree is the destructive effect of premature or excessive mental labor. I can quote you medical authority for and against every maxim of dietetics beyond the very simplest; but I defy you to find one man who ever begged, borrowed, or stole the title of M. D., and yet abused those two honorary letters by asserting, under their cover, that a child could safely study as much as a man, or that a man could safely study more than six hours a day. Most of the intelligent men in the profession would probably admit, with Scott, that even that is too large an allowance in maturity for vigorous work of the brain.

Taking, then, five hours as the reasonable daily limit of mental effort for children of eight to fourteen years, and one hour as the longest time of continuous confinement, (it was a standing rule of the Jesuits, by the way, that no pupil should study more than two hours without relaxation,) the important question now recurs, To what school shall we send Angelina?

Shall we send her, for instance, to Dothegirls' Hall? At that seminary of useful knowledge, I find by careful inquiry that the daily performance is as follows, at least in summer. The pupils rise at or before five, A. M.; at any rate, they study from five to seven, two hours. From seven to eight they breakfast. From eight to two they are in the school-room, six consecutive hours. From two to three they dine. From three to five they are "allowed" to walk or take other exercise,—that is, if it is pleasant weather, and if they feel the spirit for it, and if the time is not all used up in sewing, writing letters, school politics, and all the small miscellaneous duties of existence, for which no other moment is provided during day or night. From five to six they study; from six to seven comes the tea-table; from seven to nine study again; then bed and (at least for the stupid ones) sleep.

Eleven solid hours of study each day, Dolorosus! Eight for sleep, three for meals, two during which outdoor exercise is "allowed." There is no mistake about this statement; I wish there were. I have not imagined it; who could have done so, short of Milton and Dante, who were versed in the exploration of kindred regions of torment? But as I cannot expect the general public to believe the statement, even if you do,—and as this letter, like my previous one, may accidentally find its way into print, — and as I cannot refer to those who have personally attended the school, since they probably die off too fast to be summoned as witnesses, — I will come down to a rather milder statement, and see if you will believe that.

Shall we send her, then, to the famous New York school of Mrs. Destructive? This is recently noticed as follows in the "Household Journal": — "Of this most admirable school, for faithful and well-bred system of education, we have long intended to speak approvingly; but in the following extract from the circular the truth is more expressively given: 'From September to April the time of rising is a quarter before seven o'clock, and from April to July half an hour earlier; then breakfast; after which, from eight to nine o'clock, study, — the school opening at nine o'clock, with reading the Scriptures and prayer. From nine until half past twelve, the recitations succeed one another, with occasional short intervals of rest. From half past twelve to one, recreation and lunch. From one to three o'clock, at which hour the school closes, the studies are exclusively in the French language. . . . From three to four o'clock in the winter, but later in the summer, exercise in the open air. There are also opportunities for exercise several times in the day, at short intervals, which cannot easily be explained. From a quarter past four to five o'clock, study; then dinner, and soon after tea. From seven to nine, two hours of study; immediately after which all retire for the night, and lights in the sleeping apartments must be extinguished at half past nine.'" You have summed up the total already, Dolorosus; I see it on your lips; — nine hours and a quarter of study, and one solitary hour for exercise, not counting those inexplicable "short intervals which cannot easily be explained"!

You will be pleased to hear that I have had an opportunity of witnessing the brilliant results of Mrs. Destructive's system, in the case of my charming little neighbor, Fanny Carroll. She has lately returned from a stay of one year under that fashionable roof. In most respects, I was assured, the results of the school were all that could be desired; the mother informed me, with delight, that the child now spoke French like an angel from Paris, and handled her silver fork like a seraph from the skies. You may well suppose that I hastened to call upon her; for the gay little creature was always a great pet of mine, and I always quoted her with delight, as a proof that bloom and strength were not monopolized by English girls. In the parlor I found the mother closeted with the family physician. Soon, Fanny, aged sixteen, glided in, — a pale spectre, exquisite in costume, unexceptionable in manners, looking in all respects like an exceedingly used-up belle of five-and-twenty. "What were you just saying that some of my Fanny's symptoms were, doctor?" asked the languid mother, as if longing for a second taste of some dainty morsel. The courteous physician dropped them into her eager palm, like sugar-plums, one by one: "Vertigo, headache, neuralgic pains, and general debility." The mother sighed once genteelly at me, and then again, quite sincerely, to herself; — but I never yet saw an habitual invalid who did not seem to take a secret satisfaction in finding her child to be a chip of the old block, though both block and chip be decayed. However, nothing is now said of Miss Carroll's returning to school; and the other day I actually saw her dashing through the lane on the family pony, with a tinge of the old brightness in her cheeks. I ventured to inquire of her, soon after, if she had finished her education; and she replied, with a slight tinge of satire, that she studied regularly every day, at various "short intervals, which could not easily be explained."

Five hours a day the safe limit for study, Dolorosus, and these terrible schools quietly put into their programmes nine, ten, eleven hours; and the deluded parents think they have out-manœuvred the laws of Nature, and made a better bargain with Time. But these are private, exclusive schools, you may say, for especially favored children. We cannot afford to have most of the rising generation murdered so expensively; and in our public schools, at least, one thinks there may be some relaxation of this tremendous strain. Besides, physiological reformers had the making of our public system. "A man without high health," said Horace Mann, "is as much at war with Nature as a guilty soul is at war with the spirit of God." Look first at our Normal Schools, therefore, and see how finely their theory, also, presents this same lofty view.

"Those who have had much to do with students, especially with the female portion," said a Normal School Report a few years since, "well know the sort of martyr-spirit that extensively prevails, — how ready they often are to sacrifice everything for the sake of a good lesson, — how false are their notions of true economy in mental labor, ... sacrificing their physical natures most unscrupulously to their intellectual. Indeed, so strong had this passion for abuse become [in this institution], that no study of the laws of the physical organization, no warning, no painful experiences of their own or of their associates, were sufficient to overcome their readiness for self-sacrifice." And it appears, that, in consequence of this state of things, circulars were sent to all boarding-houses in the village, laying down stringent rules to prevent the young ladies from exceeding the prescribed amount of study.

Now turn from theory to practice. What was this "prescribed amount of study" which these desperate young females persisted in exceeding, in this model school? It began with an hour's study before daylight (in winter), — a thing most ruinous to eyesight, as multitudes have found to their cost. Then from eight to half past two, from four to half past five, from seven to nine, — with one or two slight recesses. Ten hours and three quarters daily, Dolorosus! as surely as you are a living sinner, and as surely as the Board of Education who framed that programme were sinners likewise. I believe that some Normal Schools have learned more moderation now; but I know also what forlorn wrecks of womanhood have been strewed along their melancholy history, thus far; and at what incalculable cost their successes have been purchased.

But it is premature to contemplate this form of martyrdom for Angelina, who has to run the gantlet of our common schools and high schools first. Let us consider her prospects in these, carrying with us that blessed maxim, five hours' study a day, — "Nature loves the number five," as Emerson judiciously remarks, — for our ægis against the wiles of schoolmasters.

The year 1854 is memorable for a bomb-shell then thrown into the midst of the triumphant school system of Boston, in the form of a solemn protest by the city physician against the ruinous manner in which the children were overworked. Fact, feeling, and physiology were brought to bear, with much tact and energy, and the one special point of assault was the practice of imposing out-of-school studies, beyond the habitual six hours of session. A committee of inquiry was appointed. They interrogated the grammar-school teachers. The innocent and unsuspecting teachers were amazed at the suggestion of any excess. Most of them promptly replied, in writing, that "they had never heard of any complaints on this subject from parents or guardians"; that "most of the masters were watchful upon the matter"; that "none of them *pressed* out-of-school studies"; while "the general opinion appeared to be, that a moderate amount of out-of-school study was both necessary for the prescribed course of study and wholesome in its influence on character and habits." They suggested that "commonly the ill health that might exist arose from other causes than excessive study"; one attributed it to the use of confectionery, another to fashionable parties, another to the occasional practice of "chewing pitch," — anything, everything, rather than admit that American children of fourteen could possibly be damaged by working only two hours a day *more* than Walter Scott.

However, the committee thought differently. At any rate, they fancied that they had more immediate control over the school-hours than they could exercise over the propensity of young girls for confectionery, or over the improprieties of small boys who, yet immature for tobacco, touched pitch and were defiled. So by their influence was passed that immortal Section 7 of Chapter V. of the School Regulations, — the Magna Charta of childish liberty, so far as it goes, and the only safeguard which renders it prudent to rear a family within the limits of Boston: —

"In assigning lessons to boys to be studied out of

school-hours, the instructors shall not assign a longer lesson than a boy of good capacity can acquire by an hour's study; but no out-of-school lessons shall be assigned to girls, nor shall the lessons to be studied in school be so long as to require a scholar of ordinary capacity to study out of school in order to learn them."

It appears that since that epoch this rule has "generally" been observed, "though many of the teachers would prefer a different practice." "The rule is regarded by some as an uncomfortable restriction, which without adequate reason (!) retards the progress of pupils." "A majority of our teachers would consider the permission to assign lessons for study at home to be a decided advantage and privilege." So say the later reports of the committee.

Fortunately for Angelina and the junior members of the house of Dolorosus, you are not now directly dependent upon Boston regulations. I mention them only because they represent a contest which is inevitable in every large town in the United States where the public-school system is sufficiently perfected to be dangerous. It is simply the question, whether children can bear more brain-work than men can. Physiology, speaking through my humble voice, (the personification may remind you of the days when men began poems with "Inoculation, heavenly maid!") shrieks loudly for five hours as the utmost limit, and four hours as far more reasonable than six. But even the comparatively moderate "friends of education" still claim the contrary. Mr. Bishop, the worthy Superintendent of Schools in Boston, says, (Report, 1855,) "The time daily allotted to studies may very properly be extended to seven hours a day for young persons over fifteen years of age"; and the Secretary of the Massachusetts Board of Education, in his recent volume, seems to think it a great concession to limit the period, even for younger pupils, to six.

And we must not forget, that, frame regulations as we may, the tendency will always be to overrun them. In the report of the Boston sub-committee to which I have referred, it was expressly admitted that the restrictions recommended "would not alone remedy the evil, or do much toward it; there would still be much, and with the ambitious too much, studying out of school." They ascribed the real difficulty "to the general arrangements of our schools, and to the strong pressure from various causes urging the pupils to intense application and the masters to encourage it," and said that this "could only be met by some general changes introduced by general legislation." Some few of the masters had previously admitted the same thing: "The pressure from without, the expectations of the committee, the wishes of the parents, the ambition of the pupils, and an exacting public sentiment, do tend to stimulate many to excessive application, both in and out of school."

This admits the same fact, in a different form. If these children have half their vitality taken out of them by premature and excessive brain-work, it makes no difference whether it is done in the form of direct taxation or of indirect, — whether they are compelled to it by authority or allured into it by excitement and emulation. If a horse breaks a bloodvessel by running too hard, it is no matter whether he was goaded by whip and spur, or ingeniously coaxed by the Hibernian method of a lock of hay tied six inches before his nose. The method is nothing,—it is the pace which kills. Probably the fact is, that for every extra hour directly required by the teacher, another is indirectly extorted in addition by the general stimulus of the school. The best scholars put on the added hour, because they are the best, — and the inferior scholars, because they are not the best. In either case the excess is destructive in its tendency, and the only refuge for individuals is to be found in a combination of fortunate dulness with happy indifference to shame. But is it desirable, my friend, to construct our school system on such a basis that safety and health shall be monopolized by the stupid and the shameless?

Is this magnificent system of public instruction, the glory of the world, to turn out merely a vast machine for public destruction? Look at it! as now arranged, committees are responsible to the public, teachers to committees, pupils to teachers, — all pledged to extract a maximum crop from childish brains. It is the same system of middle-men which for years ruined the Irish peasantry, with nobody ostensibly to blame. Each is responsible to the authority next above him for a certain amount, and must get it out of the victim next below him. Constant improvements in machinery perfect and expedite the work; improved gauges and meters (in the form of examinations) compute the comparative yield to a nicety, and allow no evasion. The child cannot spare an hour, for he must keep up with the other children; the teacher dares not relax, for he must keep up with the other schools; the committees must only stimulate, not check, for the eyes of the editors are upon them, and the municipal glory is at stake: every one of these, from highest to lowest, has his appointed place in the tread-mill, and must keep step with the rest; and only once a year, at the summer vacation, the vast machine stops, and the poor remains of childish brain and body are taken out and handed to anxious parents (like you, Dolorosus): —

"Here, most worthy tax-payer, is the dilapidated residue of your beloved Angelina; take her to the sea-shore for a few weeks, and make the most of her."

Do not you know that foreigners, coming from the contemplation of races less precociously intellectual, see the danger we are in, if we do not? I was struck by the sudden disappointment of an enthusiastic English teacher (Mr. Calthrop), who visited the New York schools the other day and got a little behind the scenes. "If I wanted a stranger to believe that the Millennium was not far off," he said, "I would take him to some of those grand ward-schools in New York, where able heads are trained by the thousand. I spent four or five days in doing little else than going through these truly wonderful schools. I stayed more than three hours in one of them, wondering at all I saw, admiring the stately order, the unbroken discipline of the whole arrangements, and the wonderful quickness and intelligence of the scholars. That same evening I went to see a friend, whose daughter, a child of thirteen, was at one of these schools. I examined her, and found that the little girl could hold her own with many of larger growth. 'Did she go to school to-day?' asked I. 'No,' was the answer, 'she has not been for some time, as she was beginning to get quite a serious curvature of the spine; so now she goes regularly to a gymnastic doctor.'"

I am sure that we have all had the same experience. How exciting it was, last year, to be sure, to see Angelina at the grammar-school examination, multiplying mentally 351,426 by 236,145, and announcing the result in two minutes and thirteen seconds as 82,987,492,770! I remember how you stood trembling as she staggered under the monstrous load, and how your cheek hung out the red flag of parental exultation when she came out safe. But when I looked at her colorless visage, sharp features, and shiny, consumptive skin, I groaned inwardly. It seemed as if that crop of figures, like the innumerable florets of the whiteweed, now overspreading your paternal farm, were exhausting the last atoms of vitality from a shallow soil. What a pity it is that the Deity gave to these children of ours bodies as well as brains! How it interferes with thorough instruction in the languages and the sciences! You remember the negro-trader in "Uncle Tom," who sighs for a lot of negroes specially constructed for his convenience, with the souls left out? Could not some of our school-committees take measures to secure the companion set, possessing merely the brains, and with the troublesome bodies conveniently omitted?

The truth is, that we Americans, having overcome all other obstacles to the universal education of the people, have thought to overcome even the limitations imposed by the laws of Nature; and so we were going triumphantly on, when the ruined health of our children suddenly brought us to a stand. Now we suddenly discover, that, in the absence of Inquisitions, and other unpleasant Old-World tortures, our school-houses have taken their place. We have outgrown war, we think; and yet we have not outgrown a form of contest which is undeniably more sanguinary, since one half the community actually die, under present arrangements, before they are old enough to see a battle-field, — that is, before the age of eighteen. It is an actual fact, that, if you can only keep Angelina alive up to that birthday, even if she be an ignoramus, she will at least have accomplished the feat of surviving half her contemporaries. Can there be no Peace Society to check this terrific carnage? Dolorosus, rather than have a child of mine die, as I have recently heard of a child's dying, insane from sheer overwork, and raving of algebra, I would have her come no nearer to the splendors of science than the man in the French play, who brings away from school only the general impression that two and two make five for a creditor and three for a debtor.

De Quincey wrote a treatise on "Murder considered as one of the Fine Arts," and it is certainly the fine art which receives most attention in our schools. "So far as the body is concerned," said Horace Mann of these institutions, "they provide for all the natural tendencies to physical ease and inactivity as carefully as though paleness and languor, muscular enervation and debility, were held to be constituent elements in national beauty." With this denial of the body on one side, with this tremendous stimulus of brain on the other, and with a delicate and nervous national organization to begin with, the result is inevitable. Boys hold out better than girls, partly because they are not so docile in school, partly because they are allowed to be more active out of it, and so have more recuperative power. But who has not seen some delicate girl, after five consecutive hours spent over French and Latin and Algebra, come home to swallow an indigestible dinner, and straightway settle down again to spend literally every waking hour out of the twenty-four in study, save those scanty meal-times, — protracting the labor, it may be, far into the night, till the weary eyes close unwillingly over the slate or the lexicon, — then to bed, to be vexed by troubled dreams, instead of being wrapt in the sunny slumber of childhood, — waking unrefreshed, to be reproached by parents and friends with the nervous irritability which this detestable routine has created?

For I aver that parents are more exacting than even teachers. It is outrageous to heap it all upon the pedagogues, as if they were the only apostolical successors of him whom Charles Lamb lauded, "the much calumniated good King Herod." Indeed, teachers have no objection to educating the bodies of their small subjects, if they can only be as well paid for it as for educating their intellects. But, until recently, they have never been allowed to put the bodies into the bill. And as charity begins at home, even in a physiological sense, — and as their own children's bodies required bread and butter, — they naturally postponed all regard for the physical education of their pupils until the thing acquired a marketable value. Now that the change is taking place, every schoolmaster in the land gladly adapts himself to it, and hastens to insert in his advertisement, "Especial attention given to physical education." But what good does this do, so long as parents are not willing that time enough should be deducted from the ordinary tasks to make the athletic apparatus available, — so long as it is regarded as a merit in pupils to take time from their plays and give it to extra studies, — so long as we exult over an inactive and studious child, as Dr. Beattie did over his, that "exploits of strength, dexterity, and speed" "to him no vanity or joy could bring," and then almost die of despair, like Dr. Beattie, because such a child dies before us? With girls it is far worse. "Girls, during childhood, are liable to no diseases distinct from those of boys," says Salzmann, "except the disease of education." What mother can one find in decent society, I ask you, who is not delighted to have her little girl devote even Wednesday and Saturday afternoons to additional tasks in drawing or music, rather than run the risk of having her make a noise somewhere, or possibly even soil her dress? Papa himself will far more readily appropriate ten dollars to this additional confinement, than five to the gymnasium or the riding-school. And so, beset with snares on every hand, the poor little well-educated thing can only pray the prayer recorded of a despairing child, brought up in the best society, — that she might "die and go to heaven and play with the Irish children on Saturday afternoons."

And the Sunday schools co-operate with the week-day seminaries in the pious work of destruction. Dolorosus, are all your small neighbors hard at work in committing to memory Scripture texts for a wager, — I have an impression, however, that they call it a prize, — consisting of one Bible? In my circle of society the excitement runs high. At any tea-drinking, you may hear the ladies discussing the comparative points and prospects of their various little Ellens and Harriets, with shrill eagerness; while their husbands, on the other side of the room, are debating the merits of Ethan Allen and Flora Temple, the famous trotting-horses, who are soon expected to try their speed on our "Agricultural Ground." Each horse, and each girl, appears to have enthusiastic backers, though the Sunday-school excitement has the advantage of lasting longer. From inquiry, I find the state of the field to be about as follows: — Fanny Hastings, who won the prize last year, is not to be entered for it again; she damaged her memory by the process, her teacher tells me, so that she can now scarcely fix the simplest lesson in her mind. Carry Blake had got up to five thousand verses, but had such terrible headaches that her mother compelled her to stop, some weeks ago; the texts have all vanished from her brain, but the headache unfortunately still lingers. Nelly Sanborn has reached six thousand, although her anxious father long since tried to buy her off by offering her a new Bible twice as handsome as the prize one: but what did she care for that? she said; she had handsome Bibles already, but she had no intention of being beaten by Ella Prentiss. Poor child, we see no chance for her; for Ella has it all her own way; she has made up a score of seven thousand one hundred texts, and it is only three days to the fatal Sunday. Between ourselves, I think Nelly does her work more fairly; for Ella has a marvellous ingenuity in picking out easy verses, like Jack Horner's plums, and valuing every sacred sentence, not by its subject, but by its shortness. Still, she is bound to win.

"How is her health this summer?" I asked her mother, the other day.

"Well, her verses weigh on her," said the good woman, solemnly.

And here I pledge you my word, Dolorosus, that to every one of these statements I might append, — as Miss Edgeworth does to every particularly tough story, — "*N. B. This is a fact.*" I will only add, that our Sunday-school Superintendent, who is a physician, told me that he had as strong objections to the whole thing as I could have; but that it was no use talking; all the other schools did it, and ours must; emulation was the order of the day. "Besides," he added, with that sort of cheerful hopelessness peculiar to his profession, "the boys never trouble themselves about it; and as for the girls, they would probably lose their health very soon, at any rate, and may as well devote it to a sacred cause."

Do not misunderstand me. The aim in this case is a good one, just as the aim in week-day schools is a good one, — to communicate valuable knowledge and develop the powers of the mind. The defect in policy, in both cases, appears to be, that it totally defeats its own aim, renders the employments hateful that should be delightful, and sacrifices health and joy without any adequate equivalent. All excess defeats itself. As a grown man can work more in ten hours than in fifteen, taking a series of days together, so a child can make more substantial mental progress in five hours daily than in ten. Your child's mind is not an earthen jar, to be filled by pouring into it; it is a delicate plant, to be wisely and healthfully reared; and your wife might as well attempt to enrich her mignonette-bed by laying a Greek Lexicon upon it, as try to cultivate that young nature by a top-dressing of Encyclopædias. I use the word on high authority. "Courage, my boy!" wrote Lord Chatham to his son, "only the Encyclopædia to learn!" — and the cruel diseases of a lifetime repaid Pitt for the forcing. I do not object to the severest *quality* of study for boys or girls; — while their brains work, let them work in earnest. But I do object to this immoderate and terrific *quantity*. Cut down every school, public and private, to five hours' total work *per diem* for the oldest children, and four for the younger ones, and they will accomplish more in the end than you ever saw them do in six or seven. Only give little enough at a time, and some freshness to do it with, and you may, if you like, send Angelina to any school, and put her through the whole programme of the last educational prospectus sent to me, — "Philology, Pantology, Orthology, Aristology, and Linguistics."

For what is the end to be desired? Is it to exhibit a prodigy, or to rear a noble and symmetrical specimen of a human being? Because Socrates taught that a boy who has learned to speak is not too small for the sciences, — because Tiberius delivered his father's funeral oration at the age of nine, and Marcus Aurelius put on the philosophic gown at twelve, and Cicero wrote a treatise on the art of speaking at thirteen, — because Lipsius is said to have composed a work the day he was born, meaning, say the commentators, that he began a new life at the age of ten, — because the learned Licetus, who was brought into the world so feeble as to be baked up to maturity in an oven, sent forth from that receptacle, like a loaf of bread, a treatise called "Gonopsychanthropologia," — is it, therefore, indispensably necessary, Dolorosus, that all your pale little offspring shall imitate them? Spare these innocents! it is not their fault that they are your children, — so do not visit it upon them so severely. Turn, Angelina, ever dear, and out of a little childish recreation we will yet extract a great deal of maturer wisdom for you, if we can only bring this deluded parent to his senses.

To change the sweet privilege of childhood into weary days and restless nights, — to darken its pure associations, which for many are the sole light that ever brings them back from sin and despair to the heaven of their infancy, — to banish those reveries of innocent fancy which even noisy boyhood knows, and which are the appointed guardians of its purity before conscience wakes, — to abolish its moments of priceless idleness, saturated with sunshine, blissful, aimless moments, when every angel is near, — to bring insanity, once the terrible prerogative of maturer life, down into the summer region of childhood, with blight and ruin; — all this is the work of our folly, Dolorosus, of our miserable ambition to have our unconscious little ones begin, in their very infancy, the race of desperate ambition, which has, we admit, exhausted prematurely the lives of their parents.

The worst danger of it is, that the moral is written at the end of the fable, not the beginning. The organization in youth is so dangerously elastic, that the result of these intellectual excesses is not seen until years after. When some young girl incurs spinal disease for life from some slight fall which she ought not to have felt for an hour, or some business-man breaks down in the prime of his years from some trifling over-anxiety which should have left no trace behind, the popular verdict may be, "Mysterious Providence"; but the wiser observer sees the retribution for the folly of those misspent days which enfeebled the childish constitution, instead of ripening it. One of the most admirable passages in the Report of Dr. Ray, already mentioned, is that in which he explains, that, though hard study at school is rarely the immediate cause of insanity, it is the most frequent of its ulterior causes, except hereditary tendencies. "It diminishes the conservative power of the animal economy to such a degree, that attacks of disease, which otherwise would have passed off safely, destroy life almost before danger is anticipated. Every intelligent physician understands, that, other things being equal, the chances of recovery are far less in the studious, highly intellectual child than in one of an opposite description. The immediate mischief may have seemed slight, but the brain is left in a condition of peculiar impressibility, which renders it morbidly sensitive to every adverse influence."

Indeed, here is precisely the weakness of our whole national training thus far, — brilliant immediate results, instead of wise delays. The life of the average American is a very hasty breakfast, a magnificent luncheon, a dyspeptic dinner, and no supper. Our masculine energy is, like our feminine beauty, bright and evanescent. As enthusiastic travellers inform us that there are in every American village a dozen girls of sixteen who are prettier than any English hamlet of the same size can produce, so the same village undoubtedly possesses a dozen very young men who, tried by the same standard, are "smarter" than their English compeers. Inquire again fifteen years after, when the Englishmen and Englishwomen are reported to be just in their prime, and, lo! those lovely girls are sallow old women, and the boys are worn-out men, — with fire left in them, it may be, but fuel gone, — retired from active business, very likely, and merely waiting for consumption to carry them off, as one waits for the omnibus.

To say that this should be amended is to say little. Either it must be amended, or the American race fails; — there is no middle ground. If we fail, (which I do not expect, I assure you,) we fail disastrously. If we succeed, if we bring up our vital and muscular developments into due proportion with our nervous energy, we shall have a race of men and women such as the world never saw. Dolorosus, when in the course of human events you are next invited to give a Fourth-of-July Oration, grasp at the opportunity, and take for your subject "Health." Tell your audience, when you rise to the accustomed flowers of rhetoric as the day wears on, that Health is the central luminary, of which all the stars that spangle the proud flag of our common country are but satellites; and close with a hint to the plumed emblem of our nation, (pointing to the stuffed one which will probably be exhibited on the platform,) that she should not henceforward confine her energies to the hatching of short-lived eaglets, but endeavor rather to educate a few full-grown birds.

As I take it, Nature said, some years since, — "Thus far the English is my best race; but we have had Englishmen enough; now for another turning of the globe, and a further novelty. We need something with a little more buoyancy than the Englishman; let us lighten the structure even at some peril in the process. Put in one drop more of nervous fluid and make the American." With that drop, a new range of promise opened on the human race, and a lighter, finer, more highly organized type of mankind was born. But the promise must be fulfilled through unequalled dangers. With the new drop came new intoxication, new ardors, passions, ambitions, hopes, reactions, and despairs, — more daring, more invention, more disease, more insanity, — forgetfulness, at first, of the old, wholesome traditions of living, recklessness of sin and saleratus, loss of refreshing sleep and of the power of play. To surmount all this, we have got to fight the good fight, I assure you, Dolorosus. Nature is yet pledged to produce that finer type, and if we miss it, she will leave us to decay, like our predecessors, — whirl the globe over once more, and choose a new place for a new experiment.

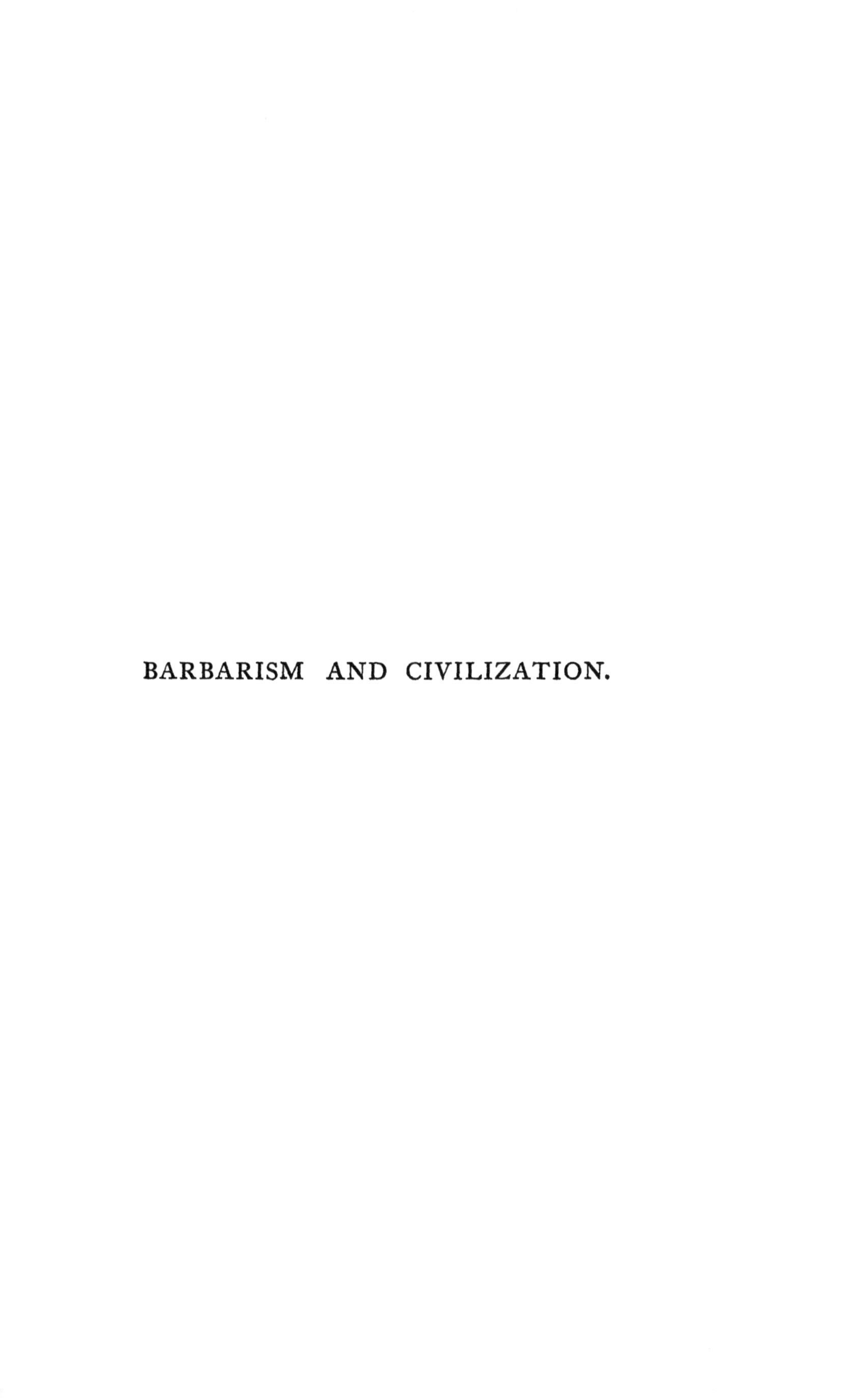

BARBARISM AND CIVILIZATION.

BARBARISM AND CIVILIZATION.

IN the interior of the island of Borneo there has been found a certain race of wild creatures, of which kindred varieties have been discovered in the Philippine Islands, in Terra del Fuego, and in Southern Africa. They walk usually almost erect upon two legs, and in that attitude measure about four feet in height; they are dark, wrinkled, and hairy; they construct no habitations, form no families, scarcely associate together, sleep in trees or in caves, feed on snakes and vermin, on ants and ants' eggs, on mice, and on each other; they cannot be tamed, nor forced to any labor; and they are hunted and shot among the trees, like the great gorillas, of which they are a stunted copy. When they are captured alive, one finds, with surprise, that their uncouth jabbering sounds like articulate language; they turn up a human face to gaze upon their captor; the females show instincts of modesty; and, in fine, these wretched beings are Men.

Men, "created in God's image," born immortal and capable of progress, and so differing from Socrates and Shakespeare only in degree. It is but a sliding scale from this melancholy debasement up to the most regal condition of humanity. A traceable line of affinity unites these outcast children with the renowned historic races of the world: the Assyrian, the Egyptian, the Ethiopian, the Jew, — the beautiful Greek, the strong Roman, the keen Arab, the passionate Italian, the stately Spaniard, the sad Portuguese, the brilliant Frenchman, the frank Northman, the wise German, the firm Englishman, and that last-born heir of Time, the American, inventor of many new things, but himself, by his temperament, the greatest novelty of all, — the American, with his cold, clear eye, his skin made of ice, and his veins filled with lava.

Who shall define what makes the essential difference between those lowest and these loftiest types? Not color; for the most degraded races seem never to be the blackest, and the builders of the Pyramids were far darker than the dwellers in the Aleutian Islands. Not unmixed purity of blood; since the Circassians, the purest type of the supreme Caucasian race, have given nothing to history but the courage of their men and the degradation of their women. Not religion; for enlightened nations have arisen under each great historic faith, while even Christianity has its Abyssinia and Arkansas. Not climate; for each quarter of the globe has witnessed both extremes. We can only say that there is an inexplicable step in progress, which we call civilization; it is the development of mankind into a sufficient maturity of strength to keep the peace and organize institutions; it is the arrival of literature and art; it is the lion and the lamb beginning to lie down together, without having, as some one has said, the lamb inside of the lion.

There are innumerable aspects of this great transformation; but there is one, in special, which has been continually ignored or evaded. In the midst of our civilization, there is a latent distrust of civilization. We are never weary of proclaiming the enormous gain it has brought to manners, to morals, and to intellect; but there is a wide-spread impression that the benefit is purchased by a corresponding physical decay. This alarm has had its best statement from Emerson. "Society never advances. It recedes as fast on one side as it gains on the other. . . . . What a contrast between the well-clad, reading, writing, thinking American, with a watch, a pencil, and a bill of exchange in his pocket, and the naked New-Zealander, whose property is a club, a spear, a mat, and the undivided twentieth part of a shed to sleep under! But compare the health of the two men, and you shall see that his aboriginal strength the white man has lost. If the traveller tell us truly, strike the savage with a broad-axe, and in a day or two the flesh shall unite and heal as if you struck the blow into soft pitch; and the same blow shall send the white man to his grave."

Were this true, the fact would be fatal. Man is a progressive being, only on condition that he begin at the beginning. He can afford to wait centuries for a brain, but he cannot subsist a second without a body. If civilization sacrifice the physical thus hopelessly to the mental, and barbarism merely sacrifice the mental to the physical, then barbarism is unquestionably the better thing, so far as it goes, because it provides the essential preliminary conditions. Barbarism is a one-story log-hut, a poor thing, but better than nothing; while such a civilization would be simply a second story, with a first story too weak to sustain it, a magnificent sky-parlor, with all heaven in view from the upper windows, but with the whole family coming down in a crash presently, through a fatal neglect of the basement. In such a view, an American Indian or a Kaffir warrior may be a wholesome object, good for something already, and for much more when he gets a brain built on. But when one sees a bookworm in his library, an anxious merchant-prince in his counting-room, tottering feebly about, his thin underpinning scarcely able to support what he has already crammed into that heavy brain of his, and he still piling in more, — one feels disposed to cry out, "Unsafe passing here! Stand from under!"

Sydney Smith, in his "Moral Philosophy," has also put strongly this case of physiological despair. "Nothing can be plainer than that a life of society is unfavorable to all the animal powers of men. . . . . A Choctaw could run from here to Oxford without stopping. I go in the mail-coach; and the time the savage has employed in learning to run so fast I have employed in learning something useful. It would not only be useless in me to run like a Choctaw, but foolish and disgraceful." But one may well suppose, that, if the jovial divine had kept himself in training for this disgraceful lost art of running, his diary might not have recorded the habit of lying two hours in bed in the morning, "dawdling and doubting," as he says, or the fact of his having "passed the whole day in an unpleasant state of body, produced by laziness"; and he might not have been compelled to invent for himself that amazing rheumatic armor, — a pair of tin boots, a tin collar, a tin helmet, and a tin shoulder-of-mutton over each of his natural shoulders, all duly filled with boiling water, and worn in patience by the sedentary Sydney.

It is also to be remembered that this statement was made in 1805, when England and Germany were both waking up to a revival of physical training, — if we may trust Sir John Sinclair in the one case, and Salzmann in the other, — such as America is experiencing now. Many years afterwards, Sydney Smith wrote to his brother, that "a working senator should lead the life of an athlete." But supposing the fact still true, that an average red man can run, and an average white man cannot, — who does not see that it is the debility, not the performance, which is discreditable? Setting aside the substantial advantages of strength and activity, there is a melancholy loss of self-respect in buying cultivation for the brain by resigning the proper vigor of the body. Let men say what they please, they all demand a life which shall be whole and sound throughout, and there is a drawback upon all gifts that are paid for in infirmities. There is no thorough satisfaction in art or intellect, if we yet feel ashamed before the Indian because we cannot run, and before the South-Sea Islander because we cannot swim. Give us a total culture, and a success without any discount of shame. After all, one feels a certain justice in Warburton's story of the Guinea trader, in Spence's Anecdotes. Mr. Pope was with Sir Godfrey Kneller one day, when his nephew, a Guinea trader, came in. "Nephew," said Sir Godfrey, "you have the honor of seeing the two greatest men in the world." "I don't know how great you may be," said the Guinea-man, "but I don't like your looks; I have often bought a man, much better than both of you together, all muscles and bones, for ten guineas."

Fortunately for the hopes of man, the alarm is unfounded. The advance of accurate knowledge dispels it. Civilization is cultivation, whole cultivation; and even in its present imperfect state, it not only permits physical training, but promotes it. The traditional glory of the savage body is yielding before medical statistics: it is becoming evident that the average barbarian, observed from the cradle to the grave, does not know enough and is not rich enough to keep his body in its highest condition, but, on the contrary, is small and sickly and short-lived and weak, compared with the man of civilization. The great athletes of the world have been civilized; the long-lived men have been civilized; the powerful armies have been civilized; and the average of life, health, size, and strength is highest to-day among those races where knowledge and wealth and comfort are most widely spread. And yet, by the common lamentation, one would suppose that all civilization is a slow suicide of the race, and that refinement and culture are to leave man at last in a condition like that of the little cherubs on old tombstones, all head and wings.

It must be owned that the delusion has all the superstitions of history in its favor, and only the facts against it. If we may trust tradition, the race has undoubtedly been tapering down from century to century since the Creation, so that the original Adam must have been more than twice the size of the Webster statue. However far back we go, admiring memory looks farther. Homer and Virgil never let their hero throw a stone without reminding us that modern heroes only live in glass houses, to have stones thrown at them. Lucretius and Juvenal chant the same lament. Xenophon, mourning the march of luxury among the Persians, says that modern effeminacy has reached such a pitch, that men have even devised coverings for their fingers, called gloves. Herodotus narrates, that, when Cambyses sent ambassadors to the Macrobians, they asked what the Persians had to eat, and how long they commonly lived. He was told that they sometimes attained the age of eighty, and that they ate a mass of crushed grain, which they termed bread. On this, they said that it was no wonder if the Persians died young, when they partook of such rubbish, and that probably they would not survive even so long, but for the wine they drank; while the Macrobians lived on flesh and milk, and survived one hundred and twenty years.

But, unfortunately, there were no Life Insurance Companies among the Macrobians, and therefore nothing to bring down this formidable average to a reliable schedule, — such as accurately informs every modern man how long he may live honestly, without defrauding either his relict or his insurers. We know, moreover, precisely what Dr. Windship can lift, at any given date, and what the rest of us cannot; but Homer and Virgil never weighed the stones which their heroes threw, nor even the words in which they described the process. It is a matter of certainty that all great exploits are severely tested by Fairbanks's scales and stop-watches. It is wonderful how many persons, in the remoter districts, assure the newspaper-editors of their ability to lift twelve hundred pounds; and many a young oarsman can prove to you that he has pulled his mile faster than Ward or Clark, if you will only let him give his own guess at time and distance.

It is easy, therefore, to trace the origin of these exaggerations. Those old navigators, for instance, who saw so many fine things which were not to be seen, how should they help peopling the barbarous realms with races of giants? Job Hartop, who three times observed a merman rise above water to his waist, near the Bermudas, — Harris, who endured such terrific cold in the Antarctics, that once, perilously blowing his nose with his fingers, it flew into the fire and was seen no more, — Knyvett, who, in the same regions, pulled off his frozen stockings, and his toes with them, but had them replaced by the ship's surgeon, — of course these men saw giants, and it is only a matter for gratitude that they vouchsafed us dwarfs also, to keep up some remains of self-respect in us. In Magellan's Straits, for instance, they saw, on one side, from three to four thousand pygmies with mouths from ear to ear; while on the other shore they saw giants whose footsteps were four times as large as an Englishman's, — which was a strong expression, considering that the Englishman's footstep had already reached round the globe.

The only way to test these earlier observations is by later ones. For instance, in the year 1772, a Dutchman named Roggewein discovered Easter Island. His expedition had cost the government a good deal, and he had to bring home his money's worth of discoveries. Accordingly, his islanders were all giants, — twice as tall, he said, as the tallest of the Europeans; "they measured, one with another, the height of twelve feet; so that we could easily, — who will not wonder at it? — without stooping, have passed between the legs of these sons of Goliah. According to their height, so is their thickness." Moreover, he "puts down nothing but the real truth, and upon the nicest inspection," and, to exhibit this caution, warns us that it would be wrong to rate the women of those regions as high as the men, they being, as he pityingly owns, "commonly not above ten or eleven feet." Sweet young creatures they must have appeared, belle and steeple in one. And it was certainly a great disappointment to Captain Cook, when, on visiting the same island, fifty years later, he could not find man or woman more than six feet tall. Thus ended the tale of this Flying Dutchman.

Thus lamentably have the inhabitants of Patagonia been also dwindling, though there, if anywhere, still lies the Cape of Bad Hope for the apostles of human degeneracy. Pigafetta originally estimated them at twelve feet. In the time of Commodore Byron, they had already grown downward; yet he said of them that they were "enormous goblins," seven feet high, every one of them. One of his officers, however, writing an independent narrative, seemed to think this a needless concession; he admits, indeed, that the women were not, perhaps, more than seven feet, or seven and a half, or, it might be, eight, "but the men were, for the most part, about nine feet high, and very often more." Lieutenant Cumming, he said, being but six feet two, appeared a mere pygmy among them. But it seems, that, in after-times, on some one's questioning this diminutive lieutenant as to the actual size of these enormous goblins, the veteran frankly confessed, that, "had it been anywhere else but in Patagonia, he should have called them good sturdy savages, and thought no more on 't."

But, these facts apart, there are certain general truths which look ominous for the reputation of the *physique* of savage tribes.

First, they cannot keep the race alive, they are always tending to decay. When first encountered by civilization, they usually tell stories of their own decline in numbers, and after that the downward movement is accelerated. They are poor, ignorant, improvident, oppressed by others' violence, or exhausted by their own; war kills them, infanticide and abortion cut them off before they reach the age of war, pestilences sweep them away, whole tribes perish by famine and small-pox. Under the stern climate of the Esquimaux and the soft skies of Tahiti, the same decline is seen. Parkman estimates that in 1763 the whole number of Indians east of the Mississippi was but ten thousand, and they were already mourning their own decay. Travellers seldom visit a savage country without remarking on the scarcity of aged people and of young children. Lewis and Clarke, Mackenzie, Alexander Henry, observed this among Indian tribes never before visited by white men; Dr. Kane remarked it among the Esquimaux, D'Azara among the Indians of South America, and many travellers in the South-Sea Islands and even in Africa, though the black man apparently takes more readily to civilization than any other race, and then develops a terrible vitality, as American politicians find to their cost.

Meanwhile, the hardships which thus decimate the tribe toughen the survivors, and sometimes give them an apparent advantage over civilized men. The savages whom one encounters are necessarily the picked men of the race, and the observer takes no census of the multitudes who have perished in the process. Civilization keeps alive, in every generation, large numbers who would otherwise die prematurely. These millions of invalids do not owe to civilization their diseases, but their lives. It is painful that your sick friend should live on Cherry Pectoral; but if he had been born in barbarism, he would neither have had it to drink nor survived to drink it.

And again, it is now satisfactorily demonstrated that these picked survivors of savage life are commonly suffering under the same diseases with their civilized compeers, and show less vital power to resist them. In barbarous nations every foreigner is taken for a physician, and the first demand is for medicines; if not the right medicines, then the wrong ones; if no medicines are at hand, the written prescription, administered internally, is sometimes found a desirable restorative. The earliest missionaries to the South-Sea Islands found ulcers and dropsy and humpbacks there before them. The English Bishop of New Zealand, landing on a lone islet where no ship had ever touched, found the whole population prostrate with influenza. Lewis and Clarke, the first explorers of the Rocky Mountains, found Indian warriors ill with fever and dysentery, rheumatism and paralysis, and Indian women in hysterics. "The toothache," said Roger Williams of the New England tribes, "is the only paine which will force their stoute hearts to cry"; even the Indian women, he says, never cry as he has heard "some of their men in this paine"; but Lewis and Clarke found whole tribes who had abolished this source of tears in the civilized manner, by having no teeth left. We complain of our weak eyes as a result of civilized habits, and Tennyson, in "Locksley Hall," wishes his children bred in some savage land, "not with blinded eyesight poring over miserable books." But savage life seems more injurious to the organs of vision than even the type of a cheap edition; for the most vigorous barbarians — on the prairies, in Southern archipelagos, on African deserts — suffer more from different forms of ophthalmia than from any other disease; without knowing the alphabet, they have worse eyes than if they were professors, and have not even the melancholy consolation of spectacles.

Again, the savage cannot, as a general rule, endure transplantation, — he cannot thrive in the country of the civilized man; whereas the latter, with time for training, can equal or excel him in strength and endurance on his own ground. As it is known that the human race generally can endure a greater variety of climate than the hardiest of the lower animals, so it is with the man of civilization, when compared with the barbarian. Kane, when he had once learned how to live in the Esquimaux country, lived better than the Esquimaux themselves; and he says expressly, that "their powers of resistance are no greater than those of well-trained voyagers from other lands." Richardson, Parkyns, Johnstone, give it as their opinion, that the European, once acclimated, bears the heat of the African deserts better than the native negro. "These Christians are devils," say the Arabs; "they can endure both cold and heat." What are the Bedouins to the Zouaves, who unquestionably would be as formidable in Lapland as in Algiers? Nay, in the very climates where the natives are fading away, the civilized foreigner multiplies; thus, the strong New-Zealanders do not average two children to a family, while the households of the English colonists are larger than at home, — which is saying a good deal.

Most formidable of all is the absence of all recuperative power in the savage who rejects civilization. No effort of will improves his condition; he sees his race dying out, and he can only drink and forget it. But the civilized man has an immense capacity for self-restoration; he can make mistakes and correct them again, sin and repent, sink and rise. Instinct can only prevent; science can cure in one generation, and prevent in the next. It is known that some twenty years ago a thrill of horror shot through all Anglo-Saxondom at the reported physical condition of the operatives in English mines and factories. It is not so generally known, that, by a recent statement of the medical inspector of factories, there is declared to have been a most astounding renovation of female health in such establishments throughout all England since that time, — the simple result of sanitary laws.

What science has done science can do. Everybody knows which symptom of American physical decline is habitually quoted as most alarming; one seldom sees a dentist who does not despair of the republic. Yet this calamity is nothing new; the elder branch of our race has been through that epidemic, and outlived it. In the robust days of Queen Bess, the teeth of the court ladies were habitually so black and decayed, that foreigners used constantly to ask if Englishwomen ate nothing but sugar. Hentzner, who visited the country in 1697, speaks of the same calamity as common among the English of all classes. Two centuries and a half have removed the stigma, — improved physical habits have put fresh pearls between the lips of all England now; and there seems no reason why we Americans may not yet be healthy, in spite of our teeth.

Thus much for general considerations; let us come now to more specific tests, beginning with the comparison of size. The armor of the knights of the Middle Ages is too small for their modern descendants: Hamilton Smith records that two Englishmen of average dimensions found no suit large enough to fit them in the great collection of Sir Samuel Meyrick. The Oriental sabre will not admit the English hand, nor the bracelet of the Kaffir warrior the English arm. The swords found in Roman tumuli have handles inconveniently small; and the great mediæval two-handed sword is now supposed to have been used only for one or two blows at the first onset, and then exchanged for a smaller one. The statements given by Homer, Aristotle, and Vitruvius represent six feet as a high standard for full-grown men; and the irrefutable evidence of the ancient door-ways, bedsteads, and tombs proves the average size of the race to have certainly not diminished in modern days. The gigantic bones have all turned out to be animal remains; even the skeleton twenty-five feet high and ten feet broad, which one *savant* wrote a book called "Gigantosteologia" to prove human, and another, a counter-argument, called "Gigantomachia," to prove animal, — neither of the philosophers taking the trouble to draw a single fragment of the fossil. The enormous savage races have turned out, as has been shown, to be travellers' tales, — even the Patagonians being brought down to an average of five feet ten inches, and being, moreover, only a part of a race, the Abipones, of which the other families are smaller. Indeed, we can all learn by our own experience how irresistible is the tendency of the imagination to attribute vast proportions to all hardy and warlike tribes. Most persons fancy the Scottish Highlanders, for instance, to have been a race of giants; yet Charles Edward was said to be taller than any man in his Highland army, and his height was but five feet nine. We have the same impression in regard to our own Aborigines. Yet, when first, upon the prairies of Nebraska, I came in sight of a tribe of genuine, unadulterated Indians, with no possession on earth but a bow and arrow and a bear-skin, — bare-skin in a double sense, I might add, — my instinctive exclamation was, "What race of dwarfs is this?" They were the descendants of the glorious Pawnees of Cooper, the heroes of every boy's imagination; yet, excepting the three chiefs, who were noble-looking men of six feet in height, the tallest of the tribe could not have measured five feet six inches.

The most careful investigations give the same results in respect to physical strength. Early travellers among our Indians, as Hearne and Mackenzie, and early missionaries to the South-Sea Islands, as Ellis, report athletic contests in which the natives could not equal the better-fed, better-clothed, better-trained Europeans. When the French *savans*, Péron, Regnier, Ransonnet, carried their dynamometers to the islands of the Indian Ocean, they found with surprise that an average English sailor was forty-two per cent stronger, and an average Frenchman thirty per cent stronger, than the strongest island tribe they visited. Even in comparing different European races, it is undeniable that bodily strength goes with the highest civilization. It is recorded in Robert Stephenson's Life, that, when the English "navvies" were employed upon the Paris and Boulogne Railway, they used spades and barrows just twice the size of those employed by their Continental rivals, and were regularly paid double. Quetelet's experiments with the dynamometer on university students showed the same results: first ranked the Englishman, then the Frenchman, then the Belgian, then the Russian, then the Southern European; for those races of Southern Europe which once ruled the Eastern and the Western worlds by physical and mental power have lost in strength as they have paused in civilization, and the easy victories of our armies in Mexico show us the result.

It is impossible to deny that the observations on this subject are yet very imperfect; and the only thing to be claimed is, that they all point one way. So far as absolute statistical tables go, the above-named French observations have till recently stood almost alone, and have been the main reliance. The just criticism has, however, been made, that the subjects of these experiments were the inhabitants of New Holland and Van Diemen's Land, by no means the strongest instances on the side of barbarism. It is, therefore, fortunate that the French tables have now been superseded by some more important comparisons, accurately made by A. S. Thomson, M. D., Surgeon of the Fifty-Eighth Regiment of the British Army, and printed in the seventeenth volume of the Journal of the London Statistical Society.

The observations were made in New Zealand, — Dr. Thomson being stationed there with his regiment, and being charged with the duty of vaccinating all natives employed by the government. The islanders thus used for experiment were to some extent picked men, as none but able-bodied persons would have been selected for employ, and as they were, moreover, (he states,) accustomed to lifting burdens, and better-fed than the majority of their countrymen. The New Zealand race, as a whole, is certainly a very favorable type of barbarism, having but just emerged from an utterly savage condition, having been cannibals within one generation, and being the very identical people among whom were recorded those wonderful cures of flesh-wounds to which Emerson has referred. Cook and all other navigators have praised their robust physical aspect, and they undoubtedly, with the Fijians and the Tongans, stand at the head of all island races. They are admitted to surpass our American Indians, as well as the Kaffirs and the Joloffs, probably the finest African races; and an accurate comparison between New-Zealanders and Anglo-Saxons will, therefore, approach as near to an *experimentum crucis* as any single set of observations can. The following tables have been carefully prepared from those of Dr. Thomson, with the addition of some scanty facts from other sources, — scanty, because, as Quetelet indignantly observes, less pains have as yet been taken to measure accurately the physical powers of man than those of any machine he has constructed or any animal he has tamed.

TABLE.

HEIGHT.	*No. measured.*	*Average.*
New-Zealanders	147	5 feet 6¾ inches.
Students at Edinburgh . .	800	5 " 7 1/10 "
Class of 1860. Cambridge (Mass.) .	106	5 " 7⅗ "
Students at Cambridge (Eng.) .	80	5 " 8⅗ "
WEIGHT.		
New-Zealanders	146	140 pounds.
Soldiers 58th Regiment . . .	1778	142 "
Class of 1860. Cambridge (Mass.) .	106	142½ "
Students at Cambridge (Eng.) . .	80	143 "
Men weighed at Boston (U. S.) Mechanics' Fair, 1860	4369	146¾ "
Englishmen (Dr. Thomson) . .	2648	148 "
Cambridge, Eng. (a newspaper statement)	——	151 "
Revolutionary officers at West Point, August 10, 1778, given in "Milledulcia," p. 273	11	226 "
AREA OF CHEST.		
New-Zealanders	151	35.36 inches.
Soldiers 58th Regiment . . .	628	35.71 "
STRENGTH IN LIFTING.		
New-Zealanders	31	367 pounds.
Students at Edinburgh, aged 25 . .	—	416 "
Soldiers 58th Regiment . . .	33	422 "

NOTE. — The range of strength among the New-Zealanders was from 250 pounds to 420 pounds; among the soldiers, from 350 pounds to 504 pounds.

But it is the test of longevity which exhibits the greatest triumph for civilization, because here the life-insurance tables furnish ample, though comparatively recent statistics. Of course, in legendary ages all lives were of enormous length; and the Hindoos in their sacred books attribute to their progenitors a career of forty million years or thereabouts, — what may safely be termed a ripe old age; for if a man were still unripe after celebrating his forty-millionth birthday, he might as well give it up. But from the beginning of accurate statistics we know that the duration of life in any nation is a fair index of its progress in civilization. Quetelet gives statistics, more or less reliable, from every nation of Northern Europe, showing a gain of ten to twenty-five per cent during the last century. Where the tables are most carefully prepared, the result is least equivocal. Thus, in Geneva, where accurate registers have been kept for three hundred years, it seems that from 1560 to 1600 the average lifetime of the citizens was twenty-one years and two months; in the next century, twenty-five years and nine months; in the century following, thirty-two years and nine months; and in the year 1833, forty years and five months; thus nearly doubling the average age of man in Geneva within those three centuries of social progress. In France, it is estimated, that, in spite of revolutions and Napoleons, human life has been gaining at the rate of two months a year for nearly a century. By a manuscript of the fourteenth century, moreover, it is shown that the rate of mortality in Paris was then one in sixteen, — one person dying annually to every sixteen of the inhabitants. It is now one in thirty-two, — a gain of a hundred per cent in five hundred years. In England the progress has been far more rapid. The rate of mortality in 1690 was one in thirty-three; in 1780 it was one in forty; and it stands now at one in sixty, — the healthiest condition in Europe, — while in half-barbarous Russia the rate of mortality is one in twenty-seven. It would be easy to multiply these statistics to any extent; but they all point one way, and no medical statistician now pretends to oppose the dictum of Hufeland, that "a certain degree of culture is physically necessary for man, and promotes duration of life."

The simple result is, that the civilized man is physically superior to the barbarian. There is now no evidence that there exists in any part of the world a savage race who, taken as a whole, surpass or even equal the Anglo-Saxon type in average physical condition; as there is also none among whom the President elect of the United States and the Commander-in-chief of his armies would not be regarded as remarkably tall men, and Dr. Windship as a remarkably strong one. "It is now well known," says Prichard, "that all savage races have less muscular power than civilized men." Johnstone in Northern Africa, and Cumming in Southern Africa, could find no one to equal them in strength of arm. At the Sandwich Islands, Ellis records, that, "when a boat manned by English seamen and a canoe with natives left the shore together, the canoe would uniformly leave the boat behind, but they would soon relax, while the seamen, pulling steadily on, would pass them, but, if the voyage took three hours, would invariably reach the destination first." Certain races may have been regularly trained by position and necessity in certain particular arts, — as Sandwich-Islanders in swimming, and our Indians in running, — and may naturally surpass the average skill of those who are comparatively out of practice in that speciality; yet it is remarkable that their greatest feats even in these ways never seem to surpass those achieved by picked specimens of civilization. The best Indian runners could only equal Lewis and Clarke's men, and Indians have been repeatedly beaten in prize-races within the last few years; while the most remarkable aquatic feat on record is probably that of Mr. Atkins of Liverpool, who recently dived to a depth of two hundred and thirty feet, reappearing above water in one minute and eleven seconds.

In the wilderness and on the prairies we find a frequent impression that cultivation and refinement must weaken the race. Not at all; they simply domesticate it. Domestication is not weakness. A strong hand does not become less muscular under a kid glove; and a man who is a hero in a red shirt will also be a hero in a white one. Civilization, imperfect as it is, has already procured for us better food, better air, and better behavior; it gives us physical training on system; and its mental training, by refining the nervous organization, makes the same quantity of muscular power go much farther. The young English ensigns and lieutenants, who at Waterloo (in the words of Wellington) "rushed to meet death as if it were a game of cricket," were the fruit of civilization. They were representatives, indeed, of the aristocracy of their nation; and here, where the aim of all institutions is to make the whole nation an aristocracy, we must plan to secure the same splendid physical superiority on a grander scale. It is in our power, by using even very moderately for this purpose our magnificent machinery of common schools, to give to the physical side of civilization an advantage which it has possessed nowhere else, not even in England or Germany. It is not yet time to suggest detailed plans on this subject, since the public mind is not yet fully awake even to the demand. When the time comes, the necessary provisions can be made easily, — at least, as regards boys; for the physical training of girls is a far more difficult problem. The organization is more delicate and complicated, the embarrassments greater, the observations less carefully made, the successes fewer, the failures far more disastrous. Any intelligent and robust man may undertake the physical training of fifty boys, however delicate their organization, with a reasonable hope of rearing nearly all of them, by easy and obvious methods, into a vigorous maturity; but what wise man or woman can expect anything like the same proportion of success, at present, with fifty American girls?

This is the most momentous health-problem with which we have to deal, — to secure the proper physical advantages of civilization for American women. Without this there can be no lasting progress. The Sandwich Island proverb says, —

> "If strong be the frame of the mother,
> Her son shall make laws for the people."

But in this country it is scarcely an exaggeration to say that every man grows to maturity surrounded by a circle of invalid female relatives, that he later finds himself the husband of an invalid wife and the parent of invalid daughters, and that he comes at last to regard invalidism, as Michelet coolly declares, the normal condition of that sex, — as if the Almighty did not know how to create a woman. This, of course, spreads a gloom over life. When I look at the morning throng of school-girls in summer, hurrying through every street, with fresh, young faces, and vesture of lilies, duly curled and straw-hatted and booted, and turned off as patterns of perfection by proud mammas, — it is not sad to me to think that all this young beauty must one day fade and die, for there are spheres of life beyond this earth, I know, and the soul is good to endure through more than one; — the sadness is in the unnatural nearness of the decay, to foresee the living death of disease that is waiting close at hand for so many, to know how terrible a proportion of those fair children are walking unconsciously into a weary, wretched, powerless, joyless, useless maturity. Among the myriad triumphs of advancing civilization, there seems but one formidable danger, and that is here.

It cannot be doubted, however, that the peril will pass by, with advancing knowledge. In proportion to our national recklessness of danger is the promptness with which remedial measures are adopted, when they at last become indispensable. In the mean time, we must look for proofs of the physical resources of woman into foreign, and even into savage lands. When an American mother tells me with pride, as occasionally happens, that her daughter can walk two miles and back without great fatigue, the very boast seems a tragedy; but when one reads that Oberea, queen of the Sandwich Islands, lifted Captain Wallis over a marsh as easily as if he had been a little child, there is a slight sense of consolation. Brunhilde, in the "Nibelungen," binds her offending lover with her girdle and slings him up to the wall. Cymburga, wife of Duke Ernest of Austria, could crack nuts between her fingers, and drive nails into a wall with her thumb; — whether she ever got her husband under it, is not recorded. Let me preserve from oblivion the renown of my Lady Butterfield, who, about the year 1700, at Wanstead, in Essex, (England,) thus advertised: — "This is to give notice to my honored masters and ladies and loving friends, that my Lady Butterfield gives a challenge to ride a horse, or leap a horse, or run afoot, or *hollo*, with any woman in England seven years younger, but not a day older, because I won't undervalue myself, being now 74 years of age." Nor should be left unrecorded the high-born Scottish damsel whose tradition still remains at the Castle of Huntingtower, in Scotland, where two adjacent pinnacles still mark the Maiden's Leap. She sprang from battlement to battlement, a distance of nine feet and four inches, and eloped with her lover. Were a young lady to go through one of our villages in a series of leaps like that, and were she to require her lovers to follow in her footsteps, it is to be feared that she would die single.

Yet the transplanted race which has in two centuries stepped from Delft Haven to San Francisco has no reason to be ashamed of its physical achievements, the more especially as it has found time on the way for one feat of labor and endurance which may be matched without fear against any historic deed. When civilization took possession of this continent, it found one vast coating of almost unbroken forest overspreading it from shore to prairie. To make room for civilization, that forest must go. What were Indians, however deadly, — what starvation, however imminent, — what pestilence, however lurking, — to a solid obstacle like this? No mere courage could cope with it, no mere subtlety, no mere skill, no Yankee ingenuity, no labor-saving machine with head for hands; but only firm, unwearying, bodily muscle to every stroke. Tree by tree, in two centuries, the forest has been felled. What were the Pyramids to that? History does not record another athletic feat so astonishing.

But there yet lingers upon this continent a forest of moral evil more formidable, a barrier denser and darker, a Dismal Swamp of inhumanity, a barbarism upon the soil, before which civilization has thus far been compelled to pause, — happy, if it could even check its spread. Checked at last, there comes from it a cry as if the light of day had turned to darkness, — when the truth simply is, that darkness is being mastered and surrounded by the light of day. Is it a good thing to "extend the area of freedom" by pillaging some feeble Mexico? and does the phrase become a bad one only when it means the peaceful progress of constitutional liberty within our own borders? The phrases which oppression teaches become the watchwords of freedom at last, and the triumph of Civilization over Barbarism is the only Manifest Destiny of America.

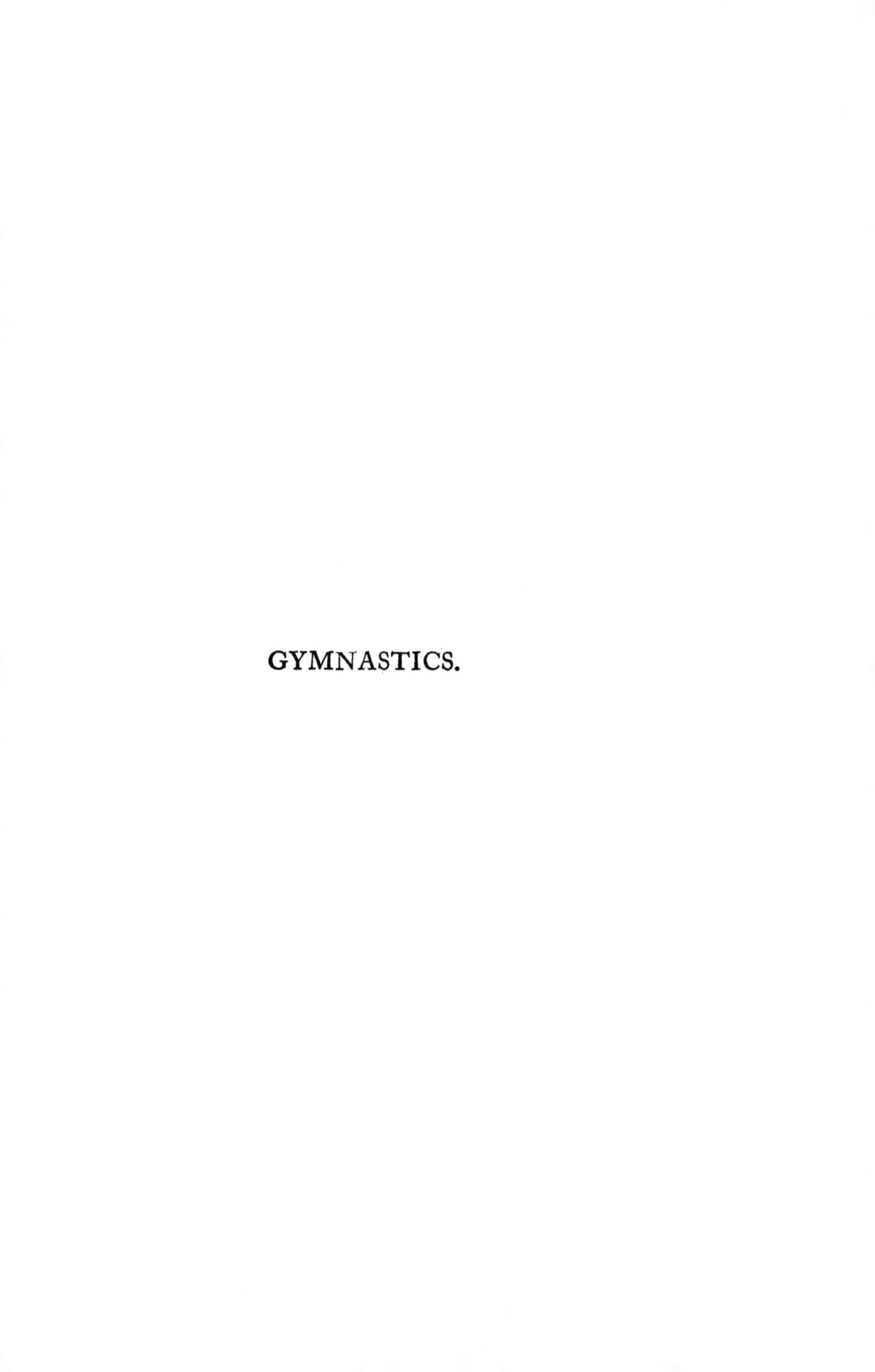

GYMNASTICS.

GYMNASTICS.

SO your zeal for physical training begins to wane a little, my friend? I thought it would, in your particular case, because it began too ardently and was concentrated too exclusively on your one hobby of pedestrianism. Just now you are literally under the weather. It is the equinoctial storm. No matter, you say; did not Olmsted foot it over all England under an umbrella? did not Wordsworth regularly walk every guest round Windermere, the day after arrival, rain or shine? So, the day before yesterday, you did your four miles out, on the Northern turnpike, and returned splashed to the waist; and yesterday you walked three miles out, on the Southern turnpike, and came back soaked to the knees. To-day the storm is slightly increasing, but you are dry thus far, and wish to remain so; exercise is a humbug; you will give it all up, and go to the Chess-Club. Don't go to the Chess-Club; come with me to the Gymnasium.

Chess may be all very well to tax with tough problems a brain otherwise inert, to vary a monotonous day with small events, to keep one awake during a sleepy evening, and to arouse a whole family next morning for the adjustment over the breakfast-table of that momentous state-question, whether the red king should have castled at the fiftieth move or not till the fifty-first. But for an average American man, who leaves his place of business at nightfall with his head a mere furnace of red-hot brains and his body a pile of burnt-out cinders, utterly exhausted in the daily effort to put ten dollars more of distance between his posterity and the poor-house, — for such a one to kindle up afresh after office-hours for a complicated chess-problem seems much as if a wood-sawyer, worn out with his week's work, should decide to order in his saw-horse on Saturday evening, and saw for fun. Surely we have little enough recreation at any rate, and, pray, let us make that little unintellectual. True, something can be said in favor of chess, — inasmuch as no money can be made out of it; but even this is not enough. For this once, lock your brains into your safe, at nightfall, with your other valuables; don't go to the Chess-Club; come with me to the Gymnasium.

Ten leaps up a steep, worn-out stairway, through a blind entry to another stairway, and yet another, and we emerge suddenly upon the floor of a large lighted room, a mere human machine-shop of busy motion, where Indian clubs are whirling, dumb-bells pounding, swings vibrating, and arms and legs flying in all manner of unexpected directions. Henderson sits with his big proportions quietly rested against the weight-boxes, pulling with monotonous vigor at the fifty-pound weights, — "the Stationary Engine" the boys call him. For a contrast, Draper is floating up and down between the parallel bars with such an airy lightness, that you think he must have hung up his body in the dressing-room, and is exercising only in his arms and clothes. Parsons is swinging in the rings, rising to the ceiling before and behind; up and down he goes, whirling over and over, converting himself into a mere tumbler-pigeon, yet still bound by the long, steady vibration of the human pendulum. Another is running a race with him, if sitting in the swing be running; and still another is accompanying their motion, clinging to the *trapèze*. Hayes, meanwhile, is spinning on the horizontal bar, now backward, now forward, twenty times without stopping, pinioned through his bent arms, like a Fakir on his iron. See how many different ways of ascending a vertical pole these boys are devising! — one climbs with hands and legs, another with hands only, another is crawling up on all-fours in Fiji fashion, while another is pegging his way up by inserting pegs in holes a foot apart, — you will see him sway and tremble yet, before he reaches the ceiling. Others are at work with a spring-board and leaping-cord; higher and higher the cord is moved, one by one the competitors step aside defeated, till the field is left to a single champion, who, like an India-rubber ball, goes on rebounding till he seems likely to disappear through the chimney, like a Ravel. Some sturdy young visitors, farmers by their looks, are trying their strength, with various success, at the sixty-pound dumb-bell, when some quiet fellow, a clerk or a tailor, walks modestly to the hundred-pound weight, and up it goes as steadily as if the laws of gravitation had suddenly shifted their course, and worked upward instead of down. Lest, however, they should suddenly resume their original bias, let us cross to the dressing-room, and, while you are assuming flannel shirt or complete gymnastic suit, as you may prefer, let us consider the merits of the Gymnasium.

Do not say that the public is growing tired of hearing about physical training. You might as well speak of being surfeited with the sight of apple-blossoms, or bored with roses, — for these athletic exercises are, to a healthy person, just as good and refreshing. Of course, any one becomes insupportable who talks all the time of this subject, or of any other; but it is the man who fatigues you, not the theme. Any person becomes morbid and tedious whose whole existence is absorbed in any one thing, be it playing or praying. Queen Elizabeth, after admiring a gentleman's dancing, refused to look at the dancing-master, who did it better. "Nay," quoth her bluff Majesty, — "'t is his business, — I 'll none of him." Professionals grow tiresome. Books are good, — so is a boat; but a librarian and a ferryman, though useful to take you where you wish to go, are not necessarily enlivening as companions. The annals of "Boxiana" and "Pedestriana" and "The Cricket-Field" are as pathetic records of monomania as the bibliographical works of Mr. Thomas Dibdin. Margaret Füller said truly, that we all delight in gossip, and differ only in the department of gossip we individually prefer; but a monotony of gossip soon grows tedious, be the theme horses or octavos.

Not one tenth-part of the requisite amount has yet been said of athletic exercises as a prescription for this community. There was a time when they were not even practised generally among American boys, if we may trust the foreign travellers of a half-century ago, and they are but just being raised into respectability among American men. Motley says of one of his Flemish heroes, that "he would as soon have foregone his daily tennis as his religious exercises," — as if ball-playing were then the necessary pivot of a great man's day. Some such pivot of physical enjoyment we must have, for no other race in the world needs it so much. Through the immense inventive capacity of our people, mechanical avocations are becoming almost as sedentary and intellectual as the professions. Among Americans, all hand-work is constantly being transmuted into brain-work; Napoleon's wish is being fulfilled, that all trades should become arts; the intellect gains, but the body suffers, and needs some other form of physical activity to restore the equilibrium. As machinery becomes perfected, all the coarser tasks are constantly being handed over to the German or Irish immigrant, — not because the American cannot do the particular thing required, but because he is promoted to something more intellectual. Thus transformed to a mental laborer, he must somehow supply the bodily deficiency. If this is true even of mechanics, it is of course true of the merchant, the student, and the professional man. The general statement recently made by Lewes, in England, certainly holds not less in America: "It is rare to meet with good digestion among the artisans of the brain, no matter how careful they may be in food and general habits. The great majority of our literary and professional men could echo the testimony of Washington Irving, if they would only indorse his wise conclusion: "My own case is a proof how one really loses by overwriting one's self and keeping too intent upon a sedentary occupation. I attribute all my present indisposition, which is losing me time, spirits, everything, to two fits of close application and neglect of all exercise while I was at Paris. I am convinced that he who devotes two hours each day to vigorous exercise will eventually gain those two and a couple more into the bargain."

Indeed, there is something involved in the matter far beyond any merely physical necessity. All our natures need something more than mere bodily exertion; they need bodily enjoyment. There is, or ought to be, in all of us a touch of untamed gypsy nature, which should be trained, not crushed. We need, in the very midst of civilization, something which gives a little of the zest of savage life; and athletic exercises furnish the means. The young man who is caught down the bay in a sudden storm, alone in his boat, with wind and tide against him, has all the sensations of a Norway sea-king, — sensations thoroughly uncomfortable, if you please, but for the thrill and glow they bring. Swim out after a storm at Dove Harbor, topping the low crests, diving through the high ones, and you feel yourself as veritable a South-Sea Islander as if you were to dine that day on missionary instead of mutton. Tramp, for a whole day, across hill, marsh, and pasture, with gun, rod, or whatever the excuse may be, and camp where you find yourself at evening, and you are as essentially an Indian on the Blue Hills as among the Rocky Mountains. Less depends upon circumstances than we fancy, and more upon our personal temperament and will. All the enjoyments of Browning's "Saul," those "wild joys of living" which make us happy with their freshness as we read of them, are within the reach of all, and make us happier still when enacted. Every one, in proportion as he develops his own physical resources, puts himself in harmony with the universe, and contributes something to it; even as Mr. Pecksniff, exulting in his digestive machinery, felt a pious delight after dinner in the thought that this wonderful apparatus was wound up and going.

A young person can no more have too much love of adventure than a mill can have too much water-power; only it needs to be worked, not wasted. Physical exercises give to energy and daring a legitimate channel, supply the place of war, gambling, licentiousness, high-way-robbery, and office-seeking. De Quincey, in like manner, says that Wordsworth made pedestrianism a substitute for wine and spirits; and Emerson thinks the force of rude periods "can rarely be compensated in tranquil times, except by some analogous vigor drawn from occupations as hardy as war." The animal energy cannot and ought not to be suppressed; if debarred from its natural channel, it will force for itself unnatural ones. A vigorous life of the senses not only does not tend to sensuality in the objectionable sense, but it helps to avert it. Health finds joy in mere existence; daily breath and daily bread suffice. This innocent enjoyment lost, the normal desires seek abnormal satisfactions. The most brutal prize-fighter is compelled to recognize the connection between purity and vigor, and becomes virtuous when he goes into training, as the heroes of old observed chastity, in hopes of conquering at the Olympic Games. The very word *ascetic* comes from a Greek word signifying the preparatory exercises of an athlete. There are spiritual diseases which coil poisonously among distorted instincts and disordered nerves, and one would be generally safer in standing sponsor for the soul of the gymnast than of the dyspeptic.

Of course, the demand of our nature is not always for continuous exertion. One does not always seek that "rough exercise" which Sir John Sinclair asserts to be "the darling idol of the English." There are delicious languors, Neapolitan reposes, Creole siestas, "long days and solid banks of flowers." But it is the birthright of the man of the temperate zones to alternate these voluptuous delights with more heroic ones, and sweeten the reverie by the toil. So far as they go, the enjoyments of the healthy body are as innocent and as ardent as those of the soul. As there is no ground of comparison, so there is no ground of antagonism. How compare a sonata and a sea-bath, or measure the Sistine Madonna against a gallop across country? The best thanksgiving for each is to enjoy the other also, and educate the mind to ampler nobleness. After all, the best verdict on athletic exercises was that of the great Sully, when he said, "I was always of the same opinion with Henry IV. concerning them: he often asserted that they were the most solid foundation, not only of discipline and other military virtues, but also of those noble sentiments and that elevation of mind which give one nature superiority over another."

We are now ready, perhaps, to come to the question, How are these athletic enjoyments to be obtained? The first and easiest answer is, By taking a long walk every day. If people would actually do this, instead of forever talking about doing it, the object might be gained. To be sure, there are various defects in this form of exercise. It is not a play, to begin with, and therefore does not withdraw the mind from its daily cares; the anxious man recurs to his problems on the way; and each mile, in that case, brings fresh weariness to brain as well as body. Moreover, there are, according to Dr. Grau, "three distinct groups of muscles which are almost totally neglected where walking alone is resorted to, and which consequently exist only in a crippled state, although they are of the utmost importance, and each stands in close *rapport* with a number of other functions of the greatest necessity to health and life." These he afterwards classifies as the muscles of the shoulders and chest, having a bearing on the lungs, — the abdominal muscles, bearing on the corresponding organs, — and the spinal muscles, which are closely connected with the whole nervous system.

But the greatest practical difficulty is, that walking, being the least concentrated form of exercise, requires a larger appropriation of time than most persons are willing to give. Taken liberally, and in connection with exercises which are more concentrated and have more play about them, it is of great value, and, indeed, indispensable. But so far as I have seen, instead of these other pursuits taking the place of pedestrianism, they commonly create a taste for it; so that, when the sweet spring days come round, you will see our afternoon gymnastic class begin to scatter literally to the four winds; or they look in for a moment, on their way home from the woods, their hands filled and scented with long wreaths of the trailing arbutus.

But the gymnasium is the normal type of all muscular exercise, — the only form of it which is impartial and comprehensive, which has something for everybody, which is available at all seasons, through all weathers, in all latitudes. All other provisions are limited: you cannot row in winter nor skate in summer, spite of parlor-skates and ice-boats; ball-playing requires comrades; riding takes money; everything needs daylight: but the gymnasium is always accessible. Then it is the only thing which trains the whole body. Military drill makes one prompt, patient, erect, accurate, still, strong. Rowing takes one set of muscles and stretches them through and through, till you feel yourself turning into one long spiral spring from finger-tips to toes. In cricket or base-ball, a player runs, strikes, watches, catches, throws, must learn quickness of hand and eye, must learn endurance also. Yet, no matter which of these may be your special hobby, you must, if you wish to use all the days and all the muscles, seek the gymnasium at last.

The history of modern gymnastic exercises is easily written: it is proper to say modern, — for, so far as apparatus goes, the ancient gymnasiums seem to have had scarcely anything in common with our own. The first institution on the modern plan was founded at Schnepfenthal, near Gotha, in Germany, in 1785, by Salzmann, a clergyman and the principal of a boys' school. After eight years of experience, his assistant, Gutsmuths, wrote a book upon the subject, which was translated into English, and published at London in 1799 and at Philadelphia in 1800, under the name of "Salzmann's Gymnastics." No similar institution seems to have existed in either country, however, till those established by Voelckers, in London, in 1824, and by Dr. Follen, at Cambridge, Mass., in 1826. Both were largely patronized at first, and died out at last. The best account of Voelckers's establishment will be found in Hone's "Every-Day Book"; its plan seems to have been unexceptionable. But Dr. James Johnson, writing his "Economy of Health" ten years after, declared that these German exercises had proved "better adapted to the Spartan youth than to the pallid sons of pampered cits, the dandies of the desk, and the squalid tenants of attics and factories," and also adds the epitaph, "This ultra-gymnastic enthusiast did much injury to an important branch of hygiene by carrying it to excess, and consequently by causing its desuetude." And Dr. Jarvis, in his "Practical Physiology," declares from personal recollection that the result of the American experiment was "general failure."

Accordingly, the English, who are reputed kings in all physical exercises, have undoubtedly been far surpassed by the Germans, and even by the French, in gymnastics. The writer of the excellent little "Handbook for Gymnastics," George Forrest, M. A., testifies strongly to this deficiency. "It is curious that we English, who possess perhaps the finest and strongest figures of all European nations, should leave ourselves so undeveloped bodily. There is not one man in a hundred who can even raise his toes to a level with his hands, when suspended by the latter members; and yet to do so is at the very beginning of gymnastic exercises. We, as a rule, are strong in the arms and legs, but weak across the loins and back, and are apparently devoid of that beautiful set of muscles that run round the entire waist, and show to such advantage in the ancient statues. Indeed, at a bathing-place, I can pick out every gymnast merely by the development of those muscles," — a statement, by the way, which has a good deal of truth in it.

It is the Germans and the military portion of the French nation, chiefly, who have developed gymnastic exercises to their present elaboration, while the working out of their curative applications was chiefly due to Ling, a Swede. In the German manuals, such, for instance, as Eiselen's "Turnübungen," are to be found nearly all the stock exercises of our institutions. Until within a few years, American skill has added nothing to these, except through the medium of the circus; but the present revival of athletic exercises is rapidly placing American gymnasts in advance of the *Turners*, both in the feats performed and in the style of doing them. Never yet have I succeeded in seeing a thoroughly light and graceful German gymnast, while again and again I have seen Americans who carried into their severest exercise such an airy, floating elegance of motion, that all the beauty of Greek sculpture appeared to return again, and it seemed as if plastic art might once more make its studio in the gymnasium.

The apparatus is not costly. Any handful of young men in the smallest country village, with a very few dollars and a little mechanical skill, can put up in any old shed or shoe-shop a few simple articles of machinery, which will, through many a winter evening, vary the monotony of the cigar and the grocery-bench by an endless variety of manly competitions. Fifteen cents will bring by mail from the publishers of the "Atlantic" Forrest's little sixpenny "Handbook," which gives a sufficient number of exercises to form an introduction to all others; and a gymnasium is thus easily established. This is just the method of the simple and sensible Ger mans, who never wait for elegant upholstery. A pair of plain parallel bars, a movable vaulting-bar, a wooden horse, a spring-board, an old mattress to break the fall, a few settees where sweethearts and wives may sit with their knitting as spectators, and there is a *Turnhalle* complete, — to be henceforward filled, two or three nights in every week, with cheery German faces, jokes, laughs, gutturals, and gambols.

But this suggests that you are being kept too long in the anteroom. Let me act as cicerone through this modest gymnastic hall of ours. You will better appreciate all this oddly-shaped apparatus, if I tell you in advance, as a connoisseur does in his picture-gallery, precisely what you are expected to think of each particular article.

You will notice, however, that a part of the gymnastic class are exercising without apparatus, in a series of rather grotesque movements which supple and prepare the body for more muscular feats: these are calisthenic exercises. Such are being at last introduced, thanks to Dr. Lewis and others, into our common schools. At the word of command, as swiftly as a conjurer twists his puzzle-paper, these living forms are shifted from one odd resemblance to another, at which it is quite lawful to laugh, especially if those laugh who win. A series of wind-mills, — a group of inflated balloons, — a flock of geese all asleep on one leg, — a circle of ballet-dancers, just poised to begin, — a band of patriots just kneeling to take an oath upon their country's altar, — a senate of tailors, — a file of soldiers, — a whole parish of Shaker worshippers, — a Japanese embassy performing *Ko-tow*: these all in turn come like shadows, so depart. This complicated attitudinizing forms the preliminary to the gymnastic hour. But now come and look at some of the apparatus.

Here is a row of Indian clubs, or sceptres, as they are sometimes called, — tapering down from giants of fifteen pounds to dwarfs of four. Help yourself to a pair of dwarfs, at first; grasp one in each hand, by the handle; swing one of them round your head quietly, dropping the point behind as far as possible, — then the other, — and so swing them alternately some twenty times. Now do the same back-handed, bending the wrist outward, and carrying the club behind the head first. Now swing them both together, crossing them in front, and then the same back-handed; then the same without crossing, and this again backward, which you will find much harder. Place them on the ground gently after each set of processes. Now, can you hold them out horizontally at arm's length, forward and then sideways? Your arms quiver and quiver, and down come the clubs thumping at last. Take them presently in a different and more difficult manner, holding each club with the point erect instead of hanging down; it tries your wrists, you will find, to manipulate them so, yet all the most graceful exercises have this for a basis. Soon you will gain the mastery of heavier implements than you begin with, and will understand how yonder slight youth has learned to handle his two heavy clubs in complex curves that seem to you inexplicable, tracing in the air a device as swift and tangled as that woven by a swarm of gossamer flies above a brook, in the sultry stillness of the summer noon.

This row of masses of iron, laid regularly in order of size, so as to resemble something between a musical instrument and a gridiron, consists of dumb-bells weighing from four pounds to a hundred. These playthings, suited to a variety of capacities, have experienced a revival of favor within a few years, and the range of exercises with them has been greatly increased. The use of very heavy ones is, so far as I can find, a peculiarly American hobby, though not originating with Dr. Windship. Even he, at the beginning of his exhibitions, used those weighing only ninety-eight pounds; and it was considered an astonishing feat, when, a little earlier, Mr. Richard Montgomery used to "put up" a dumb-bell weighing one hundred and one pounds. A good many persons, in different parts of the country, now handle one hundred and twenty-five, and Dr. Windship has got much farther on. There is, of course, a knack in using these little articles, as in every other feat, yet it takes good extensor muscles to get beyond the fifties. The easiest way of elevating the weight is to swing it up from between the knees; or it may be thrown up from the shoulder, with a simultaneous jerk of the whole body; but the only way of doing it handsomely is to put it up from the shoulder with the arm alone, without bending the knee, though you may bend the body as much as you please. Dr. Windship now puts up one hundred and forty-one pounds in this manner, and by the aid of a jerk can elevate one hundred and eighty with one arm. This particular movement with dumb-bells is most practised, as affording a test of strength; but there are many other ways of using them, all exceedingly invigorating, and all safe enough, unless the weight employed be too great, which it is very apt to be. Indeed, there is so much danger of this, that at Cambridge it has been deemed best to exclude all beyond seventy pounds. Nevertheless, the dumb-bell remains the one available form of home or office exercise: it is a whole athletic apparatus packed up in the smallest space; it is gymnastic pemmican. With one fifty-pound dumb-bell, or a pair of half that size, — or more or less, according to his strength and habits, — a man may exercise nearly every muscle in his body in half an hour, if he has sufficient ingenuity in positions. If it were one's fortune to be sent to prison, — and the access to such retirement is growing more and more facile in many regions of our common country, — one would certainly wish to carry a dumb-bell with him, precisely as Dr. Johnson carried an arithmetic in his pocket on his tour to the Hebrides, as containing the greatest amount of nutriment in the compactest form.

Apparatus for lifting is not yet introduced into most gymnasiums, in spite of the recommendations of the Roxbury Hercules: beside the fear of straining, there is the cumbrous weight and cost of iron apparatus, while, for some reason or other, no cheap and accurate dynamometer has yet come into the market. Running and jumping, also, have as yet been too much neglected in our institutions, or practised spasmodically rather than systematically. It is singular how little pains have been taken to ascertain definitely what a man can do with his body, — far less, as Quetelet has observed, than in regard to any animal which man has tamed, or any machine which he has invented. It is stated, for instance, in Walker's "Manly Exercises," that six feet is the maximum of a high leap, with a run, — and certainly one never finds in the newspapers a record of anything higher; yet it is the English tradition, that Ireland, of Yorkshire, could clear a string raised fourteen feet, and that he once kicked a bladder at sixteen. No spring-board would explain a difference so astounding. In the same way, Walker fixes the limit of a long leap without a run at fourteen feet, and with a run at twenty-two, — both being large estimates; and Thackeray makes his young Virginian jump twenty-one feet and three inches, crediting George Washington with a foot more. Yet the ancient epitaph of Phayllus the Crotonian claimed for him nothing less than fifty-five feet on an inclined plane. Certainly the story must have taken a leap also.

These ladders, aspiring indefinitely into the air, like Piranesi's stairways, are called technically peak-ladders; and dear banished T. S. K., who always was puzzled to know why Mount Washington kept up such a pique against the sky, would have found his joke fit these ladders with great precision, so frequent the disappointment they create. But try them, and see what trivial appendages one's legs may become, — since the feet are not intended to touch these polished rounds. Walk up backward on the under side, hand over hand, then forward; then go up again, omitting every other round; then aspire to the third round, if you will. Next grasp a round with both hands, give a slight swing of the body, let go, and grasp the round above with both, and so on upward; then the same, omitting one round, or more, if you can, and come down in the same way. Can you walk up on *one* hand? It is not an easy thing, but a first-class gymnast will do it, — and Dr. Windship does it, taking only every third round. Fancy a one-armed and legless hodman ascending the under side of a ladder to the roof, and reflect on the conveniences of gymnastic habits.

Here is a wooden horse; on this noble animal the Germans say that not less than three hundred distinct feats can be performed. Bring yonder spring-board, and we will try a few. Grasp these low pommels and vault over the horse, first to the right, then again to the left; then with one hand each way. Now spring to the top and stand; now spring between the hands forward, now backward; now take a good impetus, spread your feet far apart, and leap over it, letting go the hands. Grasp the pommels again and throw a somerset over it, — coming down on your feet, if the Fates permit. Now vault up and sit upon the horse, at one end, knees the same side; now grasp the pommels and whirl yourself round till you sit at the other end, facing the other way. Now spring up and bestride it; whirl round till you bestride it the other way, at the other end; do it once again, and, letting go your hand, seat yourself in the saddle. Now push away the spring-board and repeat every feat without its aid. Next, take a run and spring upon the end of the horse astride; then walk over, supporting yourself on your hands alone, the legs not touching; then backward, the same. It will be hard to balance yourself at first, and you will careen uneasily one way or the other; no matter, you will get over it somehow. Lastly, mount once more, kneel in the saddle, and leap to the ground. It appears at first ridiculously impracticable, the knees seem glued to their position, and it looks as if one would fall inevitably on his face; but falling is hardly possible. Any novice can do it, if he will only have faith. You shall learn to do it from the horizontal bar presently, where it looks much more formidable.

But first you must learn some simpler exercises on this horizontal bar: you observe that it is made movable, and may be placed as low as your knee, or higher than your hand can reach. This bar is only five inches in circumference; but it is remarkably strong and springy, and therefore we hope secure, though for some exercises our boys prefer to substitute a larger one. Try and vault it, first to the right, then to the left, as you did with the horse; try first with one hand, then see how high you can vault with both. Now vault it between your hands, forward and backward: the latter will baffle you, unless you have brought an unusual stock of India-rubber in your frame, to begin with. Raise it higher and higher, till you can vault it no longer. Now spring up on the bar, resting on your palms, and vault over from that position with a swing of your body, without touching the ground; when you have once managed this, you can vault as high as you can reach: double-vaulting this is called. Now put the bar higher than your head; grasp it with your hands, and draw yourself up till you look over it; repeat this a good many times: capital practice this, as is usually said of things particularly tiresome. Take hold of the bar again, and with a good spring from the ground try to curl your body over it, feet foremost. At first, in all probability, your legs will go angling in the air convulsively, and come down with nothing caught; but erelong we shall see you dispense with the spring from the ground and go whirling over and over, as if the bar were the axle of a wheel and your legs the spokes. Now spring upon the bar, supporting yourself on your palms, as before; put your hands a little farther apart, with the thumbs forward, then suddenly bring up your knees on the bar and let your whole body go over forward: you will not fall, if your hands have a good grasp. Try it again with your feet outside your hands, instead of between them; then once again flinging your body off from the bar and describing a long curve with it, arms stiff: this is called the Giant's Swing. Now hang to the bar by the knees,—by both knees; do not try it yet with one; then seize the bar with your hands and thrust the legs still farther and farther forward, pulling with your arms at the same time, till you find yourself sitting unaccountably on the bar itself. This our boys cheerfully denominate "skinning the cat," because the sensations it suggests, on a first experiment, are supposed to resemble those of pussy with her skin drawn over her head; but, after a few experiments, it seems like stroking the fur in the right direction, and grows rather pleasant.

Try now the parallel bars, the most invigorating apparatus of the gymnasium, and in its beginnings "accessible to the meanest capacity," since there are scarcely any who cannot support themselves by the hands on the bars, and not very many who cannot walk a few steps upon the palms, at the first trial. Soon you will learn to swing along these bars in long surges of motion, forward and backward; to go through them, in a series of springs from the hand only, without a jerk of the knees; to turn round and round between them, going forward or backward all the while; to vault over them and under them in complicated ways; to turn somersets in them and across them;

to roll over and over on them as a porpoise seems to roll in the sea. Then come the "low-standing" exercises, the grasshopper style of business; supporting yourself now with arms not straight, but bent at the elbow, you shall learn to raise and lower your body, and to hold or swing yourself as lightly in that position as if you had not felt pinioned and paralyzed hopelessly at the first trial; and whole new systems of muscles shall seem to shoot out from your shoulder-blades to enable you to do what you could not have dreamed of doing before. These bars are magical, — they are conduits of power; you cannot touch them, you cannot rest your weight on them in the slightest degree, without causing strength to flow into your body as naturally and irresistibly as water into the aqueduct-pipe when you turn it on. Do you but give the opportunity, and every pulsation of blood from your heart is pledged for the rest.

These exercises, and such as these, are among the elementary lessons of gymnastic training. Practise these thoroughly and patiently, and you will in time attain evolutions more complicated, and, if you wish, more perilous. Neglect these, to grasp at random after everything which you see others doing, and you will fail like a bookkeeper who is weak in the multiplication-table. The older you begin, the more gradual the preparation must be. A respectable middle-aged citizen, bent on improving his *physique*, goes into a gymnasium, and sees slight, smooth-faced boys going gayly through a series of exercises which show their bodies to be a triumph, not a drag, and he is assured that the same might be the case with him. Off goes the coat of our enthusiast, and in he plunges; he gripes a heavy dumb-bell and strains one shoulder, hauls at a weight-box and strains the other, vaults the bar and bruises his knee, swings in the rings once or twice till his hand slips and he falls to the floor. No matter, he thinks the cause demands sacrifices; but he subsides, for the next fifteen minutes, into more moderate exercises, which he still makes immoderate by his awkward way of doing them. Nevertheless, he goes home, cheerful under difficulties, and will try again to-morrow. To-morrow finds him stiff, lame, and wretched; he cannot lift his arm to his face to shave, nor lower it sufficiently to pull his boots on; his little daughter must help him with his shoes, and the indignant wife of his bosom must put on his hat, with that ineffectual one-sidedness to which alone the best-regulated female mind can attain, in this difficult part of costuming. His sorrows increase as the day passes; the gymnasium alone can relieve them, but his soul shudders at the remedy; and he can conceive of nothing so absurd as a second gymnastic lesson, except a first one. But had he been wise enough to place himself under an experienced adviser at the very beginning, he would have been put through a few simple movements which would have sent him home glowing and refreshed, and fancying himself half-way back to boyhood again; the slight ache and weariness of next day would have been cured by next day's exercise; and after six months' patience, by a progress almost imperceptible, he would have found himself, in respect to strength and activity, a transformed man.

Most of these discomforts, of course, are spared to boys; their frames are more elastic, and less liable to ache and strain. They learn gymnastics, as they learn everything else, more readily than their elders. Begin with a boy early enough, and if he be of a suitable temperament, he can learn in the gymnasium all the feats usually seen in the circus-ring, and could even acquire more difficult ones, if it were worth his while to try them. This is true even of the air-somersets and hand-springs which are not so commonly cultivated by gymnasts; but it is especially true of all exercises with apparatus. It is astonishing how readily our classes pick up any novelty brought into town by a strolling company, — holding the body out horizontally from an upright pole, or hanging by the back of the head, or touching the head to the heels, though this last is oftener tried than accomplished. They may be seen practising these antics, at all spare moments, for weeks, until some later hobby drives them away. From Blondin downwards, the public feats derive a large part of their wonder from the imposing height in the air at which they are done. Many a young man who can swing himself more than his own length on the horizontal ladder at the gymnasium has yet shuddered at *l'échelle périlleuse* of the Hanlons; and I noticed that even the simplest of their performances, such as holding by one hand, or hanging by the knees, seemed perfectly terrific when done at a height of twenty or thirty feet in the air, even to those who had done them a hundred times at a lower level. It was the nerve that was astounding, not the strength or skill; but the eye found it hard to draw the distinction. So when a gymnastic friend of mine, crossing the ocean lately, amused himself with hanging by one leg to the mizzen-topmast-stay, the boldest sailors shuddered, though the feat itself was nothing, save to the imagination.

Indeed, it is almost impossible for an inexperienced spectator to form the slightest opinion as to the comparative difficulty or danger of different exercises, since it is the test of merit to make the hardest things look easy.

Moreover, there may be a distinction between two feats almost imperceptible to the eye, — a change, for instance, in the position of the hands on a bar, — which may at once transform the thing from a trifle to a wonder. An unpractised eye can no more appreciate the difficulty of a gymnastic exercise by seeing it executed, than an inexperienced ear can judge of the perplexities of a piece of music by hearing it played.

The first effect of gymnastic exercise is almost always to increase the size of the arms and the chest; and new-comers may commonly be known by their frequent recourse to the tape-measure. The average increase among the students of Harvard University during the first three months of the gymnasium was nearly two inches in the chest, more than one inch in the upper arm, and more than half an inch in the fore-arm. This was far beyond what the unassisted growth of their age would account for; and the increase is always very marked for a time, especially with thin persons. In those of fuller habit the loss of flesh may counterbalance the gain in muscle, so that size and weight remain the same; and in all cases the increase stops after a time, and the subsequent change is rather in texture than in volume. Mere size is no index of strength: Dr. Windship is scarcely larger or heavier now than when he had not half his present powers.

In the vigor gained by exercise there is nothing false or morbid; it is as reliable as hereditary strength, except that it is more easily relaxed by indolent habits. No doubt it is aggravating to see some robust, lazy giant come into the gymnasium for the first time, and by hereditary muscle shoulder a dumb-bell which all your training has not taught you to handle. No matter; it is by comparing yourself with yourself that the estimate is to be made. As the writing-master exhibits with triumph to each departing pupil the uncouth copy which he wrote on entering, so it will be enough to you, if you can appreciate your present powers with your original inabilities. When you first joined the gymnastic class, you could not climb yonder smooth mast, even with all your limbs brought into service; now you can do it with your hands alone. When you came, you could not possibly, when hanging by your hands to the horizontal bar, raise your feet as high as your head,—nor could you, with any amount of spring from the ground, curl your body over the bar itself; and now you can hang at arm's length and fling yourself over it a dozen times in succession. At first, if you lowered yourself with bent elbows between the parallel bars, you could not by any manœuvre get up again, but sank to the ground a hopeless wreck; now you can raise and lower yourself an indefinite number of times. As for the weights and clubs and dumb-bells, you feel as if there must be some jugglery about them,—they have grown so much lighter than they used to be. It is you who have gained a double set of muscles to every limb; that is all. Strike out from the shoulder with your clenched hand; once your arm was loose-jointed and shaky; now it is firm and tense, and begins to feel like a natural arm. Moreover, strength and suppleness have grown together; you have not stiffened by becoming stronger, but find yourself more flexible. When you first came here, you could not touch your fingers to the ground without bending the knees, and now you can place your knuckles on the floor; then you could scarcely bend yourself backward, and now you can lay the back of your head in a chair, or walk, without crouching forward, under a bar less than three feet from the ground. You have found, indeed, that almost every feat is done originally by sheer strength, and then by agility, requiring very little expenditure of force after the precise motion is hit upon; at first labor, puffing, and a red face, — afterwards ease and the graces.

To a person who begins after the age of thirty or thereabouts, the increase of strength and suppleness, of course, comes more slowly; yet it comes as surely, and perhaps it is a more permanent acquisition, less easily lost again, than in the softer frame of early youth. There is no doubt that men of sixty have experienced a decided gain in strength and health by beginning gymnastic exercises even at that age, as Socrates learned to dance at seventy; and if they have practised similar exercises all their lives, so much is added to their chance of preserving physical youthfulness to the last. Jerome and Gabriel Ravel are reported to have spent near threescore years on the planet which their winged feet have so lightly trod; and who will dare to say how many winters have passed over the head of the still young and graceful Papanti?

Dr. Windship's most important experience is, that strength is to a certain extent identical with health, so that every increase in muscular development is an actual protection against disease. Americans, who are ashamed to confess to doing the most innocent thing for the sake of mere enjoyment, must be cajoled into every form of exercise under the plea of health. Joining, the other day, in a children's dance, I was amused by a solemn parent who turned to me, in the midst of a Virginia reel, — he still conscientious, though breathless, — and asked if I did not consider dancing to be, on the whole, a *healthy* exercise? Well, the gymnasium is healthy; but the less you dwell on that fact, the better, after you have once entered it. If it does you good, you will enjoy it; and if you enjoy it, it will do you good. With body, as with soul, the highest experience merges duty in pleasure. The better one's condition is, the less one has to think about growing better, and the more unconsciously one's natural instincts guide the right way. When ill, we eat to support life; when well, we eat because the food tastes good. It is a merit of the gymnasium, that, when properly taken, it makes one forget to think about health or anything else that is troublesome; "a man remembereth neither sorrow nor debt"; cares must be left outside, be they physical or metaphysical, like canes at the door of a museum.

No doubt, to some it grows tedious. It shares this objection with all means of exercise. To be an American is to hunger for novelty; and all instruments and appliances, especially, require constant modification: we are dissatisfied with last winter's skates, with the old boat, and with the family pony. So the zealot finds the gymnasium insufficient long before he has learned half the moves. To some temperaments it becomes a treadmill, and that, strangely enough, to diametrically opposite temperaments. A lethargic youth, requiring great effort to keep himself awake between the exercises, thinks the gymnasium slow, because he is; while an eager, impetuous young fellow, exasperated because he cannot in a fortnight draw himself up by one hand, finds the same trouble there as elsewhere, that the laws of Nature are not fast enough for his inclinations. No one without energy, no one without patience, can find permanent interest in a gymnasium; but with these qualities, and a modest willingness to live and learn, I do not see why one should ever grow tired of the moderate use of its apparatus. For one, I really never enter it without exhilaration, or leave it without a momentary regret: there are always certain special new things on the docket for trial; and when those are settled, there will be something more. It is amazing what a variety of interest can be extracted from those few bits of wood and rope and iron. There is always somebody in advance, some "man on horseback" on a wooden horse, some India-rubber hero, some slight and powerful fellow who does with ease what you fail to do with toil, some terrible Dr. Windship with an ever-waxing dumb-bell. The interest becomes semi-professional. A good gymnast enjoys going into a new and well-appointed establishment, precisely as a sailor enjoys a well-rigged ship; every rope and spar is scanned with intelligent interest; "we know the forest round us as seamen know the sea." The pupils talk gymnasium as some men talk horse. A particularly smooth and flexible horizontal pole, a desirable pair of parallel bars, a remarkably elastic spring-board, — these are matters of personal pride, and described from city to city with loving enthusiasm. The gymnastic apostle rises to eloquence in proportion to the height of the hand-swings, and points his climax to match the peak-ladders.

An objection frequently made to the gymnasium, and especially by anxious parents, is the supposed danger of accident. But this peril is obviously inseparable from all physical activity. If a man never leaves his house, the chances undoubtedly are, that he will never break his leg on the sidewalk; but if he is always to stay in the house, he might as well have no legs at all. Certainly we incur danger every time we go outside the front-door; but to remain always on the inside would prove the greatest danger of the whole. When a man slips in the street and dislocates his arm, we do not warn him against walking, but against carelessness. When a man is thrown from his horse and gratifies the surgeons by a beautiful case of compound fracture, we do not advise him to avoid a riding-school, but to go to one. Trivial accidents are not uncommon in the gymnasium, severe ones are rare, fatal ones almost unheard of,—which is far more than can be said of riding, driving, hunting, boating, skating, or even sliding down hill on a sled. Learning gymnastics is like learning to swim,—you incur a small temporary risk for the sake of acquiring powers that will lessen your risks in the end. Your increased strength and agility will carry you past many unseen perils hereafter, and the invigorated tone of your system will make accidents less important, if they happen. Some trifling sprain causes lameness for life, some slight blow brings on wasting disease, to a person whose health is merely negative, not positive,—while a well-trained frame throws it off in twenty-four hours. It is almost proverbial of the gymnasium, that it cures its own wounds.

A minor objection is, that these exercises are not performed in the open air. In summer, however, they may be, and in winter and in stormy weather it is better that they should not be. Extreme cold is not favorable to them; it braces, but stiffens; and the bars and ropes become slippery and even dangerous. In Germany it is common to have a double set of apparatus, out-doors and in-doors; and this would always be desirable, but for the increased expense. Moreover, the gymnasium should be taken in addition to out-door exercise, giving, for instance, an hour a day to each, one for training, the other for oxygen. I know promising gymnasts whose pallid complexions show that their blood is not worthy of their muscle, and they will break down. But these cases are rare, for the reason already hinted, — that nothing gives so good an appetite for out-door life as this in-door activity. It alternates admirably with skating, and seduces irresistibly into walking or rowing when spring arrives.

My young friend Silverspoon, indeed, thinks that a good trot on a fast horse is worth all the gymnastics in the world. But I learn, on inquiry, that my young friend's mother is constantly imploring him to ride in order to air her horses. It is a beautiful parental trait; but for those born horseless, what an economical substitute is the wooden quadruped of the gymnasium! Our Autocrat has well said, that the livery-stable horse is "a profligate animal"; and I do not wonder that the Centaurs of old should be suspected of having originated spurious coin. Undoubtedly it was to pay for the hire of their own hoofs.

For young men in cities, too, the facilities for exercise are limited not only by money, but by time. They must commonly take it after dark. It is in every way a blessing, when the gymnasium divides their evenings with the concert, the book, or the public meeting. Then there is no time left, and small temptation, for pleasures less pure. It gives an innocent answer to that first demand for evening excitement which perils the soul of the homeless boy in the seductive city. The companions whom he meets at the gymnasium are not the ones whose pursuits of later nocturnal hours will entice him to sin. The honest fatigue of his exercises calls for honest rest. It is the nervous exhaustion of a sedentary, frivolous, or joyless life which madly tries to restore itself by the other nervous exhaustion of debauchery. It is an old prescription, —

> "Multa tulit fecitque puer, sudavit et alsit,
> *Abstinuit venere et vino.*"

There is another class of critics whose cant is simply can't, and who, being unable or unwilling to surrender themselves to these simple sources of enjoyment, are grandiloquent upon the dignity of manhood, and the absurdity of full-grown men in playing monkey-tricks with their bodies. Full-grown men? There is not a person in the world who can afford to be a "full-grown man" through all the twenty-four hours. There is not one who does not need, more than he needs his dinner, to have habitually one hour in the day when he throws himself with boyish eagerness into interests as simple as those of boys. No church or state, no science or art, can feed us all the time; some morsels there must be of simpler diet, some moments of unadulterated play. But dignity? Alas for that poor soul whose dignity must be "preserved," — preserved in the right culinary sense, as fruits which are growing dubious in their natural state are sealed up in jars to make their acidity presentable! "There 's beggary in the love that can be reckoned," and degradation in the dignity that has to be preserved. Simplicity is the only dignity. If one has not the genuine article, no affluence of starch, no snow-drift of white-linen decency, will furnish any substitute. If one has it, he will retain it, whether he stand on his head or his heels. Nothing is really undignified but affectation or conceit; and for the total extinction and annihilation of every vestige of these, there are few things so effectual as athletic exercises.

Still another objection is that of the medical men, that

the gymnasium, as commonly used, is not a specific prescription for the special disease of the patient. But setting aside the claims of the system of applied gymnastics, which Ling and his followers have so elaborated, it is enough to answer, that the one great fundamental disorder of all Americans is simply nervous exhaustion, and that for this the gymnasium can never be misdirected, though it may be used to excess. Of course one can no more cure overwork of brain by overwork of body, than one can restore a wasted candle by lighting it at the other end. But by subtracting an hour a day from the present amount of purely intellectual fatigue, and inserting that quantum of bodily fatigue in its place, you begin an immediate change in your conditions of life. Moreover, the great object is not merely to get well, but to keep well. The exhaustion of overwork can almost always be cured by a water-cure, or by a voyage, which is a salt-water cure; but the problem is, how to make the whole voyage of life perpetually self-curative. Without this, there is perpetual dissatisfaction and chronic failure. Emerson well says, "Each class fixes its eye on the advantages it has not, — the refined on rude strength, the democrat on birth and breeding." This is the aim of the gymnasium, to give to the refined this rude strength, or its better substitute, refined strength. It is something to secure to the student or the clerk the strong muscles, hearty appetite, and sound sleep of the sailor and the ploughman, — to enable him, if need be, to out-row the fisherman, and outrun the mountaineer, and lift more than his porter, and to remember headache and dyspepsia only as he recalls the primeval whooping-cough of his childhood. I am one of those who think that the Autocrat rides his hobby of the pavements a little too far; but it is useless to deny, that, within the last few years of gymnasiums and boat-clubs, the city has been gaining on the country in physical development. Here in our town we had all the city and college boys assembled in July to see the regattas, and all the country-boys in September to see the thousand-dollar base-ball match; and it was impossible to deny, whatever one's theories, that the guests of the regatta showed the finer *physique*.

The secret is, that, though the country offers to farmers more oxygen than is accessible to anybody in the city, yet not all dwellers in the country are farmers, and even this favored class suffer from other causes, being usually the very last to receive those lessons of food and clothing and bathing and ventilation which have their origin in cities. Physical training is not a mechanical, but a vital process: no bricks without straw; no good *physique* without good materials and conditions. The farmer knows, that, to rear a premium colt or calf, he must oversee every morsel that it eats, every motion it makes, every breath it draws, — must guard against over-work and under-work, cold and heat, wet and dry. He remembers it for the quadrupeds, but he forgets it for his children, his wife, and himself: so his cattle deserve a premium, and his family does not.

Neglect is the danger of the country; the peril of the city is in living too fast. All mental excitement acts as a stimulant, and, like all stimulants, debilitates when taken in excess. This explains the unnatural strength and agility of the insane, always followed by prostration; and even moderate cerebral excitement produces similar results, so far as it goes. Quetelet discovered that sometimes after lecturing, or other special intellectual action, he could perform gymnastic feats impossible to him at other times. The fact is unquestionable; and it is also certain that an extreme in this direction has precisely the contrary effect, and is fatal to the physical condition. One may spring up from a task of moderate mental labor with a sense of freedom, like a bow let loose; but after an immoderate task one feels like the same bow too long bent, flaccid, nerveless, all the elasticity gone. Such fatigue is far more overwhelming than any mere physical exhaustion. I have lounged into the gymnasium, after an afternoon's skating, supposing myself quite tired, and have found myself in excellent condition; and I have gone in after an hour or two of some specially concentrated anxiety or thought, without being aware that the body was at all fatigued, and found it good for nothing. Such experiences are invaluable; all the libraries cannot so illustrate the supremacy of immaterial forces. Thought, passion, purpose, expectation, absorbed attention even, all feed upon the body's powers; let them act one atom too intensely, or one moment too long, and this wondrous physical organization finds itself drained of its forces to support them. It does not seem strange that strong men should have died by a single ecstasy of emotion too convulsive, when we bear within us this tremendous engine whose slightest pulsation so throbs in every fibre of our frame.

The relation between mental culture and physical powers is a subject of the greatest interest, as yet but little touched, because so few of our physiologists have been practical gymnasts. Nothing is more striking than the tendency of all athletic exercises, when brought to perfection, to eliminate mere brute bulk from the competition, and give the palm to more subtile qualities, agility, quickness, a good eye, a ready hand, — in short, superior fineness of organization. Any clown can learn the military manual exercise; but it needs brain-power to drill with the Zouaves. Even a prize-fight tests strength less than activity and "science." The game of base-ball, as played in our boyhood, was a simple, robust, straightforward contest, where the hardest hitter was the best man; but it is every year becoming perfected into a sleight-of-hand, like cricket; mere strength is now almost valueless in playing it, and it calls rather for the qualities of the billiard-player. In the last champion-match at Worcester, nearly the whole time was consumed in skilful feints and parryings, and it took five days to make fifty runs. And these same characteristics mark gymnastic exercises above all; men of great natural strength are very apt to be too slow and clumsy for them, and the most difficult feats are usually done by persons of comparatively delicate *physique* and a certain artistic organization. It is this predominance of the nervous temperament which is yet destined to make American gymnasts the foremost in the world....

Indeed, the gymnasium is as good a place for the study of human nature as any. The perpetual analogy of mind and body can be appreciated only where both are trained with equal system. In both departments the great prizes are not won by the most astounding special powers, but by a certain harmonious adaptation. There is a physical tact, as there is a mental tact. Every process is accomplished by using just the right stress at just the right moment; but no two persons are alike in the length of time required for these little discoveries. Gymnastic genius lies in gaining at the first trial what will cost weeks of perseverance to those less happily gifted. And as the close, elastic costume which is worn by the gymnast, or should be worn, allows no merit or defect of figure to be concealed, so the close contact of emulation exhibits all the varieties of temperament. One is made indolent by success, and another is made ardent; one is discouraged by failure, and another aroused by it; one does everything best the first time and slackens ever after, while another always begins at the bottom and always climbs to the top.

One of the most enjoyable things in these mimic emulations is this absolute genuineness in their gradations of success. In the great world outside, there is no immediate and absolute test for merit. There are cliques and puffings and jealousies, quarrels of authors, tricks of trade, caucusing in politics, hypocrisy among the deacons. We distrust the value of others' successes, they distrust ours, and we all sometimes distrust our own. There are those who believe in Shakespeare, and those who believe in Tupper. All merit is measured by sliding scales, and each has his own theory of the sliding. In a dozen centuries it will all come right, no doubt. In the mean time there is vanity in one half the world, and vexation of spirit in the other half, and each man joins each half in turn. But once enter the charmed gate of the gymnasium, and you leave shams behind. Though you be saint or sage, no matter, the inexorable laws of gravitation are around you. If you flinch, you fail; if you slip, you fall. That bar, that rope, that weight, shall test you absolutely. Can you handle it, it is well; but if not, stand aside for him who can. You may have every other gift and grace, it counts for nothing; he, not you, is the man for the hour. The code of Spanish aristocracy is slight and flexible compared with this rigid precedence. It is Emerson's Astræa; each registers himself, and there is no appeal. No use to kick and struggle, no use to apologize; do not say that to-night you are tired, last night you felt ill. These excuses may serve for a day, but no longer. A slight margin is allowed for moods and variations, but it is not great after all. One revels in this Palace of Truth: defeat itself is a satisfaction, before a tribunal of such absolute justice.

This contributes to that healthful ardor with which, in these exercises, a man forgets the things which are behind and presses forward to fresh achievements. This perpetually saves from vanity; for everything seems a trifle, when you have once attained to it. The aim which yesterday filled your whole gymnastic horizon you overtake and pass as a boat passes a buoy: until passed, it was an absorbing goal; when passed, a mere speck in the distance. Yesterday you could swing yourself three rounds upon the horizontal ladder; to-day, after weeks of effort, you have suddenly attained to the fourth, and instantly all that long laborious effort vanishes, to be formed again between you and the fifth round: five, five is the only goal for heroic labor to-day; and when five is attained, there will be six, and so on while the Arabic numerals hold out. A childish aim, no doubt; but is not this what we all recognize as the privilege of childhood, to obtain exaggerated enjoyment from little things? When you have come to the really difficult feats of the gymnasium, — when you have conquered the "barber's curl" and the "peg-pole," — when you can draw yourself up by one arm, and perform the "giant's swing" over and over, without changing hands, and vault the horizontal bar as high as you can reach it, — when you can vault across the high parallel bars between your hands backward, or walk through them on your palms with your feet in the vicinity of the ceiling, — then you will reap the reward of your past labors, and may begin to call yourself a gymnast.

It is pleasant to think, that, so great is the variety of exercises in the gymnasium, even physical deficiencies and deformities do not wholly exclude from its benefits. I have seen an invalid girl, so lame from childhood that she could not stand without support, whose general health had been restored, and her bust and arms made a study for a sculptor, by means of gymnastics. Nay, there are odd compensations of Nature by which even exceptional formations may turn to account in athletic exercises. A squinting eye is a treasure to a boxer, a left-handed batter is a prize in a cricketing eleven, and one of the best gymnasts in Chicago is an individual with a wooden leg, which he takes off at the commencement of affairs, thus economizing weight and stowage, and performing achievements impossible except to unipeds.

In the enthusiasm created by this emulation, there is necessarily some danger of excess. Dr. Windship approves of exercising only every other day in the gymnasium; but as most persons take their work in a more diluted form than his, they can afford to repeat it daily, unless warned by headache or languor that they are exceeding their allowance. There is no good in excess; our constitutions cannot be hurried. The law is universal, that exercise strengthens as long as nutrition balances it, but afterwards wastes the very forces it should increase. We cannot make bricks faster than Nature supplies us with straw.

It is one good evidence of the increasing interest in these exercises, that the American gymnasiums built during the past year or two have far surpassed all their predecessors in size and completeness, and have probably no superiors in the world. The Seventh Regiment Gymnasium in New York, just opened by Mr. Abner S. Brady, is one hundred and eighty feet by fifty-two, in its main hall, and thirty-five feet in height, with nearly a thousand pupils. The beautiful hall of the Metropolitan Gymnasium, in Chicago, measures one hundred and eight feet by eighty, and is twenty feet high at the sides, with a dome in the centre, forty feet high, and the same in diameter. Next to these probably rank the new gymnasium at Cincinnati, the Tremont Gymnasium at Boston, and the Bunker Hill Gymnasium at Charlestown, all recently opened. Of college institutions the most complete are probably those at Cambridge and New Haven, — the former being eighty-five feet by fifty, and the latter one hundred feet by fifty, in external dimensions. The arrangements for instruction are rather more systematic at Harvard, but Yale has several valuable articles of apparatus — as the rack-bars and the series of rings — which have hardly made their appearance, as yet, in Massachusetts, though considered indispensable in New York institutions.

Gymnastic exercises are as yet but very sparingly introduced into our seminaries, primary or professional, though a great change is already beginning. Until lately all our educational plans have assumed man to be a merely sedentary being; we have employed teachers of music and drawing to go from school to school to teach those elegant arts, but have had none to teach the art of health. Accordingly, the pupils have exhibited more complex curves in their spines than they could possibly portray on the blackboard, and acquired such discords in their nervous systems as would have utterly disgraced their singing. It is something to have got beyond the period when active sports were actually prohibited. I remember when there was but one boat owned by a Cambridge student, and that was soon reported to have been suppressed by the Faculty, on the plea that there was a college law against a student's keeping domestic animals, and a boat was a domestic animal within the meaning of the statute. Manual labor was thought less reprehensible; but schools on this basis have never yet proved satisfactory, because either the hands or the brains have always come off second-best from the effort to combine: it is a law of Nature, that after a hard day's work one does not need more work, but play. But in many of the German common schools one or two hours are given daily to gymnastic exercises with apparatus, with sometimes the addition of Wednesday or Saturday afternoon; and this was the result, as appears from Gutsmuth's book, of precisely the same popular reaction against a purely intellectual system which is visible in our community now. In the French military school at Joinville, the degree of Bachelor of Agility is formally conferred; but Horace Mann's remark still holds good, that it is seldom thought necessary to train men's bodies for any purpose except to destroy those of other men. However, in view of the present wise policy of our leading colleges, we shall have to stop croaking before long, especially as enthusiastic alumni already begin to fancy a visible improvement in the *physique* of graduating classes on Commencement Day.

It would be unpardonable, in this connection, not to speak a good word for the favorite hobby of the day, — Dr. Lewis, and his system of gymnastics, or, more properly, of calisthenics. Dr. Windship had done all that was needed in apostleship of severe exercises, and there was wanting some man with a milder hobby, perfectly safe for a lady to drive. The Fates provided that man, also, in Dr. Lewis, — so hale and hearty, so profoundly confident in the omnipotence of his own methods and the uselessness of all others, with such a ready invention, and such an inundation of animal spirits that he could flood any company, no matter how starched or listless, with an unbounded appetite for ball-games and bean-games. How long it will last in the hands of others than the projector remains to be seen, especially as some of his feats are more exhausting than average gymnastics; but, in the mean time, it is just what is wanted for multitudes of persons who find or fancy the real gymnasium to be unsuited to them. It will especially render service to female pupils, so far as they practise it; for the accustomed gymnastic exercises seem never yet to have been rendered attractive to them, on any large scale, and with any permanency. Girls, no doubt, learn as readily as boys to row, to skate, and to swim, — any muscular inferiority being perhaps counterbalanced in swimming by their greater physical buoyancy, in skating by their dancing-school experience, and in rowing by their music-lessons enabling them more promptly to fall into regular time, — though these suggestions may all be fancies rather than facts. The same points help them, perhaps, in the lighter calisthenic exercises; but when they come to the apparatus, one seldom sees a girl who takes hold like a boy: it, perhaps, requires a certain ready capital of muscle, at the outset, which they have not at command, and which it is tedious to acquire afterwards. Yet there seem to be some cases, as with the classes of Mrs. Molineaux at Cambridge, where a good deal of gymnastic enthusiasm is created among female pupils, and it may be, after all, that the deficiency lies thus far in the teachers.

Experience is already showing that the advantages of school-gymnasiums go deeper than was at first supposed. It is not to be the whole object of American education to create scholars or idealists, but to produce persons of a solid strength, — persons who, to use the most expressive Western phrase that ever was coined into five monosyllables, "will do to tie to"; whereas to most of us it would be absurd to tie anything but the Scriptural millstone. In the military school of Brienne, the only report appended to the name of the little Napoleon Bonaparte was "Very healthy"; and it is precisely his class of boys for whom there is least place in a purely intellectual institution. A child of immense animal activity and unlimited observing faculties, personally acquainted with every man, child, horse, dog, in the township, — intimate in the families of oriole and grasshopper, pickerel and turtle, — quick of hand and eye, — in short, born for practical leadership and victory, — such a boy finds no provision for him in most of our seminaries, and must, by his constitution, be either truant or torment. The theory of the institution ignores such aptitudes as his, and recognizes no merits save those of some small sedentary linguist or mathematician, — a blessing to his teacher, but an object of watchful anxiety to the family physician, and whose career is endangering not only his health, but his humility. Introduce now some athletic exercises as a regular part of the school-drill, instantly the rogue finds his legitimate sphere, and leads the class; he is no longer an outcast, no longer has to look beyond the school for companions and appreciation; while, on the other hand, the youthful pedant, no longer monopolizing superiority, is brought down to a proper level. Presently comes along some finer fellow than either, who cultivates all his faculties, and is equally good at spring-board and blackboard; and straightway, since every child wishes to be a Crichton, the whole school tries for the combination of merits, and the grade of the juvenile community is perceptibly raised.

What is true of childhood is true of manhood also. What a shame it is that even Kingsley should fall into the cant of deploring maturity as a misfortune, and declaring that our freshest pleasures come "before the age of fourteen"! Health is perpetual youth, — that is, a state of positive health. Merely negative health, the mere keeping out of the hospital for a series of years, is not health. Health is to feel the body a luxury, as every vigorous child does, — as the bird does when it shoots and quivers through the air, not flying for the sake of the goal, but for the sake of the flight, — as the dog does when he scours madly across the meadow, or plunges into the muddy blissfulness of the stream. But neither dog nor bird nor child enjoys his cup of physical happiness — let the dull or the worldly say what they will — with a felicity so cordial as the educated palate of conscious manhood. To "feel one's life in every limb," this is the secret bliss of which all forms of athletic exercise are merely varying disguises; and it is absurd to say that we cannot possess this when character is mature, but only when it is half developed. As the flower is better than the bud, so should the fruit be better than the flower.

We need more examples of a mode of living which shall not alone be a success in view of some ulterior object, but which shall be, in its nobleness and healthfulness, successful every moment as it passes on. Navigating a wholly new temperament through history, this American race must of course form its own methods and take nothing at second-hand; but the same triumphant combination of bodily and mental training which made human life beautiful in Greece, strong in Rome, simple and joyous in Germany, truthful and brave in England, must yet be moulded to a higher quality amid this varying climate and on these low shores. The regions of the world most garlanded with glory and romance, Attica, Provence, Scotland, were originally more barren than Massachusetts; and there is yet possible for us such an harmonious mingling of refinement and vigor, that we may more than fulfil the world's expectation, and may become classic to ourselves.

A NEW COUNTERBLAST.

A NEW COUNTERBLAST.

"He that taketh tobacco saith he cannot leave it, it doth bewitch him." — KING JAMES'S *Counterblast to Tobacco.*

AMERICA is especially responsible to the whole world for tobacco, since the two are twin-sisters, born to the globe in a day. The sailors first sent on shore by Columbus came back with news of a new continent and a new condiment. There was solid land, and there was a novel perfume, which rolled in clouds from the lips of the natives. The fame of the two great discoveries instantly began to overspread the world; but the smoke travelled fastest, as is its nature. There are many races which have not yet heard of America: there are very few which have not yet tasted of tobacco. A plant which was originally the amusement of a few savage tribes has become in a few centuries the fancied necessary of life to the most enlightened nations of the earth, and it is probable that there is nothing cultivated by man which is now so universally employed.

And the plant owes this width of celebrity to a combination of natural qualities so remarkable as to yield great diversities of good and evil fame. It was first heralded as a medical panacea, "the most sovereign and precious weed that ever the earth tendered to the use of man," and was seldom mentioned, in the sixteenth century, without some reverential epithet. It was a plant divine, a canonized vegetable. Each nation had its own pious name to bestow upon it. The French called it *herbe sainte, herbe sacrée, herbe propre à tous maux, panacée antarctique,* — the Italians, *herba santa croce,* — the Germans, *heilig wundkraut.* Botanists soberly classified it as *herba panacea* and *herba sancta,* and Gerard in his "Herbal" fixed its name finally as *sana sancta Indorum,* by which title it commonly appears in the professional recipes of the time. Spenser, in his "Faërie Queene," bids the lovely Belphœbe gather it as "divine tobacco," and Lilly the Euphuist calls it "our holy herb Nicotian," ranking it between violets and honey. It was cultivated in France for medicinal purposes solely, for half a century before any one there used it for pleasure, and till within the last hundred years it was familiarly prescribed, all over Europe, for asthma, gout, catarrh, consumption, headache; and, in short, was credited with curing more diseases than even the eighty-seven which Dr. Shew now charges it with producing.

So vast were the results of all this sanitary enthusiasm, that the use of tobacco in Europe probably reached its climax in a century or two, and has since rather diminished than increased, in proportion to the population. It probably appeared in England in 1586, being first used in the Indian fashion, by handing one pipe from man to man throughout the company; the medium of communication being a silver tube for the higher classes, and a straw and walnut-shell for the baser sort. Paul Hentzner, who travelled in England in 1598, and Monsieur Misson, who wrote precisely a century later, note almost in the same words "a perpetual use of tobacco"; and the latter suspects that this is what makes "the generality of Englishmen so taciturn, so thoughtful, and so melancholy." In Queen Elizabeth's time, the ladies of the court "would not scruple to blow a pipe together very socially." In 1614 it was asserted that tobacco was sold openly in more than seven thousand places in London, some of these being already attended by that patient Indian who still stands seductive at tobacconists' doors. It was also estimated that the annual receipts of these establishments amounted to more than three hundred thousand pounds. Elegant ladies had their pictures painted, at least one in 1650 did, with pipe and box in hand. Rochefort, a rather apocryphal French traveller in 1672, reported it to be the general custom in English homes to set pipes on the table in the evening for the females as well as males of the family, and to provide children's luncheon-baskets with a well-filled pipe, to be smoked at school, under the directing eye of the master. In 1703, Lawrence Spooner wrote that "the sin of the kingdom in the intemperate use of tobacco swelleth and increaseth so daily, that I can compare it to nothing but the waters of Noah, that swelled fifteen cubits above the highest mountains." The deluge reached its height in England — so thinks the amusing and indefatigable Mr. Fairholt, author of "Tobacco and its Associations" — in the reign of Queen Anne. Steele, in the "Spectator," (1711,) describes the snuff-box as a rival to the fan among ladies; and Goldsmith pictures the belles at Bath as entering the water in full bathing costume, each provided with a small floating basket, to hold a snuff-box, a kerchief, and a nosegay. And finally, in 1797, Dr. Clarke complains of the handing about of the snuff-box in churches during worship, "to the great scandal of religious people," — adding, that kneeling in prayer was prevented by the large quantity of saliva ejected in all directions. In view of such formidable statements as these, it is hardly possible to believe that the present generation surpasses or even equals the past in the consumption of tobacco.

And all this sudden popularity was in spite of a vast persecution which sought to unite all Europe against this indulgence, in the seventeenth century. In Russia, its use was punishable with amputation of the nose; in Berne, it ranked next to adultery among offences; Sandys, the traveller, saw a Turk led through the streets of Constantinople mounted backward on an ass with a tobacco-pipe thrust through his nose. Pope Urban VIII., in 1624, excommunicated those who should use it in churches, and Innocent XII., in 1690, echoed the same anathema. Yet within a few years afterwards travellers reported that same free use of snuff in Romish worship which still astonishes spectators. To see a priest, during the momentous ceremonial of High Mass, enliven the occasion by a voluptuous pinch, is a sight even more astonishing, though perhaps less disagreeable, than the well-used spittoon which decorates so many Protestant pulpits.

But the Protestant pulpits did their full share in fighting the habit, for a time at least. Among the Puritans, no man could use tobacco publicly, on penalty of a fine of two and sixpence, or in a private dwelling, if strangers were present; and no two could use it together. That iron pipe of Miles Standish, still preserved at Plymouth, must have been smoked in solitude, or not at all. This strictness was gradually relaxed, however, as the clergy took up the habit of smoking; and I have seen an old painting, on the panels of an ancient parsonage in Newburyport, representing a jovial circle of portly divines sitting pipe in hand around a table, with the Latin motto,

"In essentials unity, in non-essentials liberty, in all things charity." Apparently the tobacco was one of the essentials, since there was unity respecting that. Furthermore, Captain Underhill, hero of the Pequot War, boasted to the saints of having received his assurance of salvation "while enjoying a pipe of that good creature, tobacco," "since when he had never doubted it, though he should fall into sin." But it is melancholy to relate that this fall did presently take place, in a very flagrant manner, and brought discredit upon tobacco conversions, as being liable to end in smoke.

Indeed, some of the most royal wills that ever lived in the world have measured themselves against the tobacco-plant and been defeated. Charles I. attempted to banish it, and in return the soldiers of Cromwell puffed their smoke contemptuously in his face, as he sat a prisoner in the guard-chamber. Cromwell himself undertook it, and Evelyn says that the troopers smoked in triumph at his funeral. Wellington tried it, and the artists caricatured him on a pipe's head with a soldier behind him defying with a whiff that imperial nose. Louis Napoleon is said to be now attempting it, and probably finds his subjects more ready to surrender the freedom of the press than of the pipe.

The more recent efforts against tobacco, like most arguments in which morals and physiology are mingled, have lost much of their effect through exaggeration. On both sides there has been enlisted much loose statement, with some bad logic. It is, for instance, unreasonable to hold up the tobacco-plant to general indignation because Linnæus classed it with the natural order *Luridæ*, — since he attributed the luridness only to the color of those plants, not to their character. It is absurd to denounce it as belonging to the poisonous nightshade tribe, when the potato and the tomato also appertain to that perilous domestic circle. It is hardly fair even to complain of it for yielding a poisonous oil, when these two virtuous plants — to say nothing of the peach and the almond — will, under sufficient chemical provocation, do the same thing. Two drops of nicotine will, indeed, kill a rabbit; but so, it is said, will two drops of solanine. Great are the resources of chemistry, and a well-regulated scientific mind can detect something deadly almost anywhere.

Nor is it safe to assume, as many do, that tobacco predisposes very powerfully to more dangerous dissipations. The non-smoking Saxons were probably far more intemperate in drinking than the modern English; and Lane, the best authority, points out that wine is now far less used by the Orientals than at the time of the "Arabian Nights," when tobacco had not been introduced. And in respect to yet more perilous sensual excesses, tobacco is now admitted, both by friends and foes, to be quite as much a sedative as a stimulant.

The point of objection on the ground of inordinate expense is doubtless better taken, and can be met only by substantial proof that the enormous outlay is a wise one. Tobacco may be "the anodyne of poverty," as somebody has said, but it certainly promotes poverty. This narcotic lulls to sleep all pecuniary economy. Every pipe may not, indeed, cost so much as that jewelled one seen by Dibdin in Vienna, which was valued at a thousand pounds; or even as the German meerschaum which was passed from mouth to mouth through a whole regiment of soldiers till it was colored to perfection, having never been allowed to cool, — a bill of one hundred pounds being ultimately rendered for the tobacco consumed. But how heedlessly men squander money on this pet luxury! By the report of the English University Commissioners, some ten years ago, a student's annual tobacco-bill often amounts to forty pounds. Dr. Solly puts thirty pounds as the lowest annual expenditure of an English smoker, and knows many who spend one hundred and twenty pounds, and one three hundred pounds a year, on tobacco alone. In this country the facts are hard to obtain, but many a man smokes twelve four-cent cigars a day, and many a man four twelve-cent cigars, — spending in either case about half a dollar a day and not far from two hundred dollars per annum. An industrious mechanic earns his two dollars and fifty cents a day, or a clerk his eight hundred dollars a year, spends a quarter of it on tobacco, and *the rest* on his wife, children, and miscellaneous expenses.

But the impotency which marks some of the stock arguments against tobacco extends to most of those in favor of it. My friend assures me that every one needs some narcotic, that the American brain is too active, and that the influence of tobacco is quieting, — great is the enjoyment of a comfortable pipe after dinner. I grant, on observing him at that period, that it appears so. But I also observe, that, when the placid hour has passed away, his nervous system is more susceptible, his hand more tremulous, his temper more irritable on slight occasions, than during the days when the comfortable pipe chances to be omitted. The only effect of the narcotic appears, therefore, to be a demand for another narcotic; and there seems no decided advantage over the life of the birds and bees, who appear to keep their nervous systems in tolerably healthy condition with no narcotic at all.

The argument drawn from a comparison of races is no

better. Germans are vigorous and Turks are long-lived, and they are all great smokers. But certainly the Germans do not appear so vivacious, nor the Turks so energetic, as to afford triumphant demonstrations in behalf of the sacred weed. Moreover, the Eastern tobacco is as much milder than ours, as are the Continental wines than even those semi-alcoholic mixtures which prevail at scrupulous communion-tables. And as for German health, Dr. Schneider declares, in the London "Lancet," that it is because of smoke that all his educated countrymen wear spectacles, that an immense amount of consumption is produced in Germany by tobacco, and that English insurance companies are proverbially cautious in insuring German lives. Dr. Carlyon gives much the same as his observation in Holland. These facts may be overstated, but they are at least as good as those which they answer.

Not much better is the excuse alleged in the social and genial influences of tobacco. It certainly seems a singular way of opening the lips for conversation by closing them on a pipe-stem, and it would rather appear as if Fate designed to gag the smokers and let the non-smokers talk. But supposing it otherwise, does it not mark a condition of extreme juvenility in our social development, if no resources of intellect can enable a half-dozen intelligent men to be agreeable to each other, without applying the forcing process, by turning the room into an imperfectly organized chimney? Brilliant women can be brilliant without either wine or tobacco, and Napoleon always maintained that without an admixture of feminine wit conversation grew tame. Are all male beings so much stupider by nature than the other sex, that men require stimulants and narcotics to make them mutually endurable?

And as the conversational superiorities of woman disprove the supposed social inspirations of tobacco, so do her more refined perceptions yet more emphatically pronounce its doom. Though belles of the less mature description, eulogistic of sophomores, may stoutly profess that they dote on the Virginian perfume, yet cultivated womanhood barely tolerates the choicest tobacco-smoke, even in its freshness, and utterly recoils from the stale suggestions of yesterday. By whatever enthusiasm misled, she finds something abhorrent in the very nature of the thing. In vain did loyal Frenchmen baptize the weed as the queen's own favorite, *Herba Catherinæ Medicæ;* it is easier to admit that Catherine de' Medici was not feminine than that tobacco is. Man also recognizes the antagonism; there is scárcely a husband in America who would not be converted from smoking, if his wife resolutely demanded her right of moiety in the cigar-box. No Lady Mary, no loveliest Marquise, could make snuff-taking beauty otherwise than repugnant to this generation. Rustic females who habitually chew even pitch or spruce-gum are rendered thereby so repulsive that the fancy refuses to pursue the horror farther and imagine it tobacco; and all the charms of the veil and the fan can scarcely reconcile the most fumacious American to the *cigarrito* of the Spanish fair. How strange seems Parton's picture of General Jackson puffing his long clay pipe on one side of the fireplace and Mrs. Jackson puffing hers on the other! No doubt, to the heart of the chivalrous backwoodsman those smoke-dried lips were yet the altar of early passion, — as that rather ungrammatical tongue was still the music of the spheres; but the unattractiveness of that conjugal counterblast is Nature's own protest against smoking.

The use of tobacco must, therefore, be held to mark a rather coarse and childish epoch in our civilization, if nothing worse. Its most ardent admirer hardly paints it into his picture of the Golden Age. It is difficult to associate it with one's fancies of the noblest manhood, and Miss Muloch reasonably defies the human imagination to portray Shakespeare or Dante with pipe in mouth. Goethe detested it; so did Napoleon, save in the form of snuff, which he apparently used on Talleyrand's principle, that diplomacy was impossible without it. Bacon said, "Tobacco-smoking is a secret delight, serving only to steal away men's brains." Newton abstained from it: the contrary is often claimed, but thus says his biographer, Brewster, — saying that "he would make no necessities to himself." Franklin says he never used it, and never met with one of its votaries who advised him to follow the example. John Quincy Adams used it in early youth, and after thirty years of abstinence said, that, if every one would try abstinence for three months, it would annihilate the practice, and add five years to the average length of human life.

In attempting to go beyond these general charges of waste and foolishness, and to examine the physiological results of the use of tobacco, one is met by the contradictions and perplexities which haunt all such inquiries. Doctors, of course, disagree, and the special cases cited triumphantly by either side are ruled out as exceptional by the other. It is like the question of the precise degree of injury done by alcoholic drinks. To-day's newspaper writes the eulogy of A. B., who recently died at the age of ninety-nine, without ever tasting ardent spirits; to-morrow's will add the epitaph of C. D., aged one hundred, who has imbibed a quart of rum a day since reaching the age of indiscretion; and yet, after all, both editors have to admit that the drinking usages of society are growing decidedly more decent. It is the same with the tobacco argument. Individual cases prove nothing either way; there is such a range of vital vigor in different individuals, that one may withstand a life of error, and another perish in spite of prudence. The question is of the general tendency. It is not enough to know that Dr. Parr smoked twenty pipes in an evening, and lived to be seventy-eight; that Thomas Hobbes smoked thirteen, and survived to ninety-two; that Brissiac of Trieste died at one hundred and sixteen, with a pipe in his mouth; and that Henry Hartz of Schleswig used tobacco steadily from the age of sixteen to one hundred and forty-two; nor would any accumulation of such healthy old sinners prove anything satisfactory. It seems rather overwhelming, to be sure, when Mr. Fairholt assures us that his respected father "died at the age of seventy-two: he had been twelve hours a day in a tobacco-manufactory for nearly fifty years; and he both smoked and chewed while busy in the labors of the workshop, sometimes in a dense cloud of steam from drying the damp tobacco over the stoves; and his health and appetite were perfect to the day of his death: he was a model of muscular and stomachic energy; in which his son, who neither smokes, snuffs, nor chews, by no means rivals him." But until we know precisely what capital of health the venerable tobacconist inherited from his fathers, and in what condition he transmitted it to his sons, the statement certainly has two edges.

For there are facts equally notorious on the other side. It is not denied that it is found necessary to exclude tobacco, as a general rule, from insane asylums, or that it produces, in extreme cases, among perfectly sober persons, effects akin to delirium tremens. Nor is it denied that terrible local diseases follow it, — as, for instance, cancer of the mouth, which has become, according to the eminent surgeon, Brouisson, the disease most dreaded in the French hospitals. He has performed sixty-eight operations for this, within fourteen years, in the Hospital St. Eloi, and traces it entirely to the use of tobacco. Such facts are chiefly valuable as showing the tendency of the thing. Where the evils of excess are so glaring, the advantages of even moderate use are questionable. Where weak persons are made insane, there is room for suspicion that the strong may suffer unconsciously. You may say that the victims must have been constitutionally nervous; but where is the native-born American who is not?

In France and England the recent inquiries into the effects of tobacco seem to have been a little more systematic than our own. In the former country, the newspapers state, the attention of the Emperor was called to the fact that those pupils of the Polytechnic School who used this indulgence were decidedly inferior in average attainments to the rest. This is stated to have led to its prohibition in the school, and to the forming of an anti-tobacco organization, which is said to be making great progress in France. I cannot, however, obtain from any of our medical libraries any satisfactory information as to the French agitation, and am led by private advices to believe that even these general statements are hardly trustworthy. The recent English discussions are, however, more easy of access.

"The Great Tobacco Question," as the controversy in England was called, originated in a Clinical Lecture on

Paralysis, by Mr. Solly, Surgeon of St. Thomas's Hospital, which was published in the "Lancet," December 13, 1856. He incidentally spoke of tobacco as an important source of this disease, and went on to say: "I know of no single vice which does so much harm as smoking. It is a snare and a delusion. It soothes the excited nervous system at the time, to render it more irritable and feeble ultimately. It is like opium in this respect; and if you want to know all the wretchedness which this drug can produce, you should read the 'Confessions of an English Opium-Eater.'" This statement was presently echoed by J. Ranald Martin, an eminent surgeon, "whose Eastern experience rendered his opinion of immense value," and who used language almost identical with that of Mr. Solly: — "I can state of my own observation, that the miseries, mental and bodily, which I have witnessed from the abuse of cigar-smoking, far exceed anything detailed in the 'Confessions of an Opium-Eater.'"

This led off a controversy, which continued for several months, in the columns of the "Lancet," — a controversy conducted in a wonderfully good-natured spirit, considering that more than fifty physicians took part in it, and that these were almost equally divided. The debate took a wide range, and some interesting facts were elicited: as that Lord Raglan, General Markham, and Admirals Dundas and Napier always abandoned tobacco from the moment when they were ordered on actual service; that nine tenths of the first-class men at the Universities were non-smokers; that two Indian chiefs told Power, the actor, that "those Indians who smoked gave out soonest in the chase"; and so on. There were also American examples, rather loosely gathered: thus, a remark of the venerable Dr. Waterhouse, made many years ago, was cited as the contemporary opinion of "the Medical Professor in Harvard University"; also it was mentioned, as an acknowledged fact, that the American *physique* was rapidly deteriorating because of tobacco, and that coroners' verdicts were constantly being thus pronounced on American youths: "Died of excessive smoking." On the other hand, that eminent citizen of our Union, General Thomas Thumb, was about that time professionally examined in London, and his verdict on tobacco was quoted to be, that it was "one of his chief comforts"; also mention was made of a hapless quack who announced himself as coming from Boston, and who, to keep up the Yankee reputation, issued a combined advertisement of "medical advice gratis" and "prime cigars."

But these stray American instances were of course quite outnumbered by the English, and there is scarcely an ill which was not in this controversy charged upon tobacco by its enemies, nor a physical or moral benefit which was not claimed for it by its friends. According to these, it prevents dissension and dyspnœa, inflammation and insanity, saves the waste of tissue and of time, blunts the edge of grief, and lightens pain. "No man was ever in a passion with a pipe in his mouth." There are more female lunatics chiefly because the fumigatory education of the fair sex has been neglected. Yet it is important to notice that these same advocates almost outdo its opponents in admitting its liability to misuse, and the perilous consequences. "The injurious effects of excessive smoking," — "there is no more pitiable object than the inveterate smoker," — "sedentary life is incompatible with smoking," — highly pernicious, — general debility, — secretions all wrong, — cerebral softening, — partial paralysis, — trembling of the hand, — enervation and depression, — great irritability, — neuralgia, — narcotism of the heart: this Chamber of Horrors forms a part of the very Temple of Tobacco, as builded, not by foes, but by worshippers. "All men of observation and experience," they admit, "must be able to point to instances of disease and derangement from the abuse of this luxury." Yet they advocate it, as the same men advocate intoxicating drinks; not meeting the question, in either case, whether it be wise, or even generous, for the strong to continue an indulgence which is thus confessedly ruinous to the weak.

The controversy had its course, and ended, like most controversies, without establishing anything. The editor of the "Lancet," to be sure, summed up the evidence very fairly, and it is worth while to quote him: "It is almost unnecessary to make a separate inquiry into the pathological conditions which follow upon excessive smoking. Abundant evidence has been adduced of the gigantic evils which attend the abuse of tobacco. Let it be granted at once that there is such a thing as moderate smoking, and let it be admitted that we cannot accuse tobacco of being guilty of the whole of Cullen's 'Nosology'; it still remains that there is a long catalogue of frightful penalties attached to its abuse." He then proceeds to consider what is to be called abuse: as, for instance, smoking more than one or two cigars or pipes daily, — smoking too early in the day or too early in life, — and in general, the use of tobacco by those with whom it does not agree, — which rather reminds one of the early temperance pledges, which bound a man to drink no more rum than he found to be good for him. But the Chief Justice of the Medical Court finally instructs his jury of readers that young men should give up a dubious pleasure for a certain good, and abandon tobacco altogether: "Shun the habit of smoking as you would shun self-destruction. As you value your physical and moral well-being, avoid a habit which for you can offer no advantage to compare with the dangers you incur."

Yet, after all, neither he nor his witnesses seem fairly to have hit upon what seem to this present writer the two incontrovertible arguments against tobacco; one being drawn from theory, and the other from practice.

First, as to the theory of the thing. The laws of Nature warn every man who uses tobacco for the first time, that he is dealing with a poison. Nobody denies this attribute of the plant; it is "a narcotic poison of the most active class." It is not merely that a poison can by chemical process be extracted from it, but it is a poison in its simplest form. Its mere application to the skin has often produced uncontrollable nausea and prostration. Children have in several cases been killed by the mere application of tobacco ointment to the head. Soldiers have simulated sickness by placing it beneath the armpits, — though in most cases our regiments would probably consider this a mistaken application of the treasure. Tobacco, then, is simply and absolutely a poison.

Now to say that a substance is a poison, is not to say that it inevitably kills; it may be apparently innocuous, if not incidentally beneficial. King Mithridates, it is said, learned habitually to consume these dangerous commodities; and the scarcely less mythical Du Chaillu, after the fatigues of his gorilla warfare, found decided benefit from two ounces of arsenic. But to say that a substance is a poison, is to say at least that it is a noxious drug, — that it is a medicine, not an aliment, — that its effects are pathological, not physiological, — and that its use should therefore be exceptional, not habitual. Not tending to the preservation of a normal state, but at best to the correction of some abnormal one, its whole value, if it have any, lies in the rarity of its application. To apply a powerful drug at a certain hour every day, is like a schoolmaster's whipping his pupil at a certain hour every day: the victim may become inured, but undoubtedly the specific value of the remedy must vanish with the repetition.

Thus much would be true, were it proved that tobacco is in some cases apparently beneficial. No drug is beneficial, when constantly employed. But, furthermore, if not beneficial, it then is injurious. As Dr. Holmes has so forcibly expounded, every medicine is in itself hurtful. All noxious agents, according to him, cost a patient, on an average, five per cent of his vital power; that is, twenty times as much would kill him. It is believed that they are sometimes indirectly useful; it is known that they are always directly hurtful. That is, I have a neighbor on one side who takes tobacco to cure his dyspepsia, and a neighbor on the other side who takes blue pill for his infirmities generally. The profit of the operation may be sure or doubtful; the outlay is certain, and to be deducted in any event. I have no doubt, my dear Madam, that your interesting son has learned to smoke, as he states, in order to check that very distressing toothache which so hindered his studies; but I sincerely think it would be better to have the affliction removed by a dentist at a cost of fifty cents, than by a drug at an expense of five per cent of vital power.

Fortunately, when it comes to the practical test, the whole position is conceded to our hands, and the very devotees of tobacco are false to their idol. It is not merely that the most fumigatory parent dissuades his sons from the practice; but there is a more remarkable instance. If any two classes can be singled out in the community as the largest habitual consumers of tobacco, it must be the college students and the the city "roughs" or "rowdies," or whatever the latest slang name is, — for these roysterers, like oysters, incline to names with an *r* in. Now the "rough," when brought to a physical climax, becomes the prize-fighter; and the college student is seen in his highest condition as the prize-oarsman; and both these representative men, under such circumstances of ambition, straightway abandon tobacco. Such a concession, from such a quarter, is worth all the denunciations of good Mr. Trask. Appeal, O anxious mother! from Philip smoking to Philip training. What your progeny will not do for any considerations of ethics or economy, — to save his sisters' olfactories or the atmosphere of the family altar, — that he does unflinchingly at one word from the stroke-oar or the commodore. In so doing, he surrenders every inch of the ground, and owns unequivocally that he is in better condition without tobacco. The old traditions of training are in some other respects being softened: strawberries are no longer contraband, and the last agonies of thirst are no longer a part of the prescription; but training and tobacco are still incompatible. There is not a regatta or a prize-fight in which the betting would not be seriously affected by the discovery that either party used the beguiling weed.

The argument is irresistible, — or rather, it is not so much an argument as a plea of guilty under the indictment. The prime devotees of tobacco voluntarily abstain from it, like Lord Raglan and Admiral Napier, when they wish to be in their best condition. But are we ever, any of us, in too good condition? Have all the sanitary conventions yet succeeded in detecting one man, in our high-pressure America, who finds himself too well? If a man goes into training for the mimic contest, why not for the actual one? If he needs steady nerves and a cool head for the play of life, — and even prize-fighting is called "sporting," — why not for its earnest? Here we are all croaking that we are not in the health in which our twentieth birthday found us, and yet we will not condescend to the wise abstinence which even twenty practises. Moderate training is simply a rational and healthful life.

So palpable is this, that there is strong reason to believe that the increased attention to physical training is operating against tobacco. If we may trust literature, as has been shown, its use is not now so great as formerly, in spite of the vague guesses of alarmists. "It is estimated," says Mr. Coles, "that the consumption of tobacco in this country is eight times as great as in France and three times as great as in England, in proportion to the population"; but there is nothing in the world more uncertain than "It is estimated." It is frequently estimated, for instance, that nine out of ten of our college students use tobacco; and yet, by the statistics of the last graduating class at Cambridge, it appears that it is used by only thirty-one out of seventy-six. I am satisfied that the extent of the practice is often exaggerated. In a gymnastic club of young men, for instance, where I have had opportunity to take the statistics, it is found that less than one quarter use it, though there has never been any agitation or discussion of the matter. These things indicate that it can no longer be claimed, as Molière asserted two centuries ago, that he who lives without tobacco is not worthy to live.

And as there has been some exaggeration in describing the extent to which Tobacco is King, so there has doubtless been some overstatement as to the cruelty of his despotism. Enough, however, remains to condemn him. The present writer, at least, has the firmest conviction, from personal observation and experience, that the imagined benefits of tobacco-using (which have never, perhaps, been better stated than in an essay which appeared in the Atlantic Monthly, in August, 1860) are ordinarily an illusion, and its evils a far more solid reality, — that it stimulates only to enervate, soothes only to depress, — that it neither permanently calms the nerves nor softens the temper nor enlightens the brain, but that in the end its tendencies are precisely the opposites of these, beside the undoubted incidental objections of costliness and uncleanness. When men can find any other instance of a poisonous drug which is suitable for daily consumption, they will be more consistent in using this. When it is admitted to be innocuous to those who are training for athletic feats, it may be possible to suppose it beneficial to those who are out of training. Meanwhile there seems no ground for its supporters except that to which the famous Robert Hall was reduced, as he says, by "the Society of Doctors of Divinity." He sent a message to Dr. Clarke, in return for a pamphlet against tobacco, that he could not possibly refute his arguments and could not possibly give up smoking.

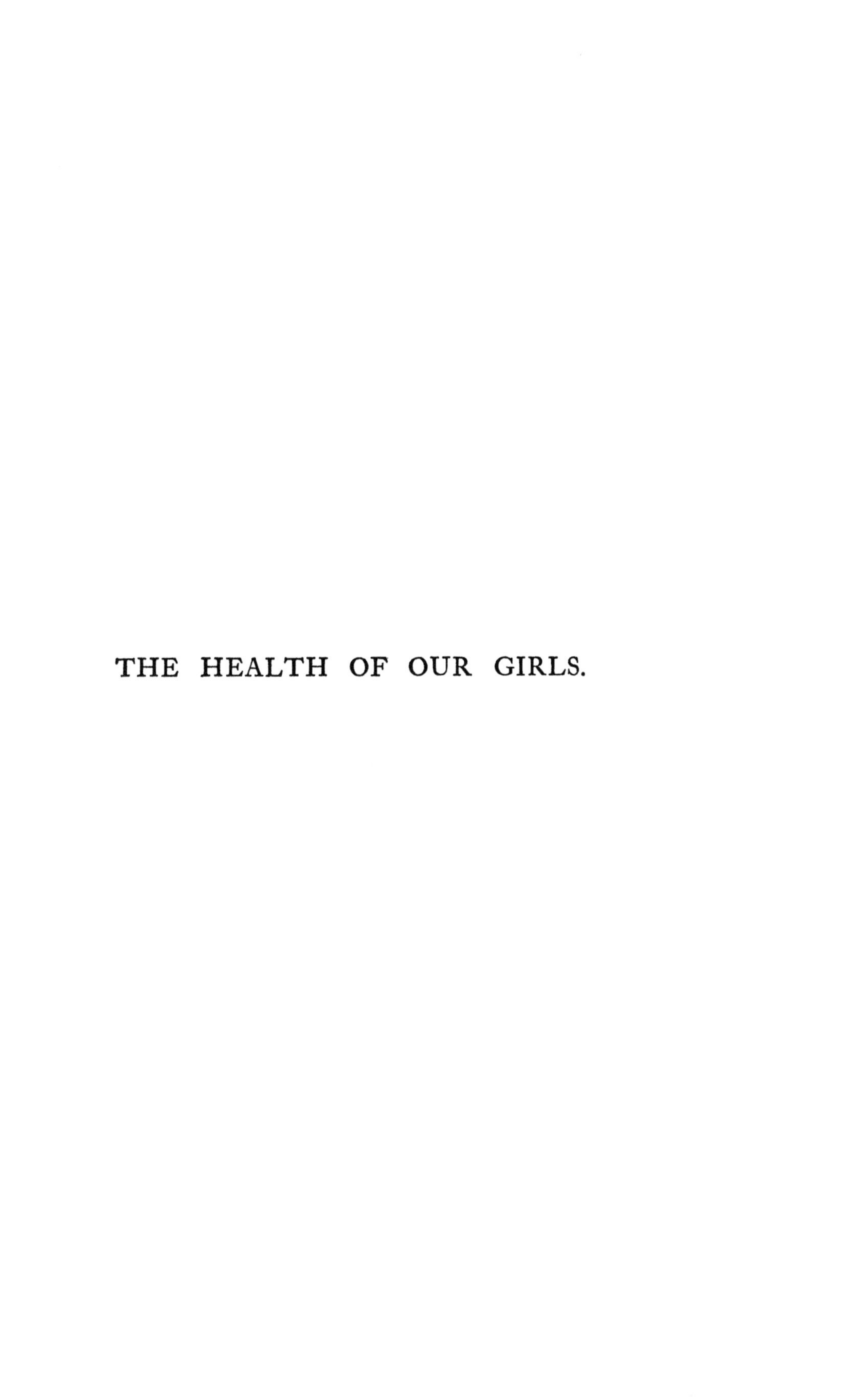

THE HEALTH OF OUR GIRLS.

THE HEALTH OF OUR GIRLS.

AMONG the lower animals, so far as the facts have been noticed, there seems no great inequality, as to strength or endurance, between the sexes. In migratory tribes, as of birds or buffaloes, the males are not observed to slacken or shorten their journeys from any gallant deference to female weakness, nor are the females found to perish disproportionately through exhaustion. It is the English experience, that among coursing-dogs and race-horses there is no serious sexual inequality. Ælian says that Semiramis did not exult when in the chase she captured a lion, but was proud when she took a lioness, the dangers of the feat being far greater. Hunters as willingly encounter the male as the female of most savage beasts; and if an adventurous fowler, plundering an eagle's nest, has his eyes assaulted by the parent-bird, it is no matter whether the discourtesy proceeds from the gentleman or the lady of the household.

Passing to the ranks of humanity, it is the general rule, that, wherever the physical nature has a fair chance, the woman shows no extreme deficiency of endurance or strength. Even the sentimental physiology of Michelet is compelled to own that his elaborate theories of lovely invalidism have no application to the peasant-women of

France, that is, to nineteen twentieths of the population. Among human beings, the disparities of race and training far outweigh those of sex. The sedentary philosopher, turning from his demonstration of the hopeless inferiority of woman, finds with dismay that his Irish or negro handmaiden can lift a heavy coal-hod more easily than he. And while the dream is vanishing of the superiority of savage races on every other point, it still remains unquestionable that in every distinctive attribute of physical womanhood the barbarian has the advantage.

The truth is, that in all countries female health and strength go with peasant habits. In Italy, for instance, About says, that, of all useful animals, the woman is the one that the Roman peasant employs with the most profit. "She makes the bread and the cake of Turkish corn; she spins, she weaves, she sews; she goes every day three miles for wood and a mile for water; she carries on her head the load of a mule; she toils from sunrise to sunset without resisting or even complaining. The children, which she brings forth in great numbers, and which she nurses herself, are a great resource; from the age of four years they can be employed in guarding other animals."

Beside this may be placed the experience of Moffat, the African missionary, who, seeing a party of native women engaged in their usual labor of house-building, and just ready to put the roof on, suggested that some of the men who stood by should lend a hand. It was received with general laughter; but Mahuto, the queen, declared that the plan, though hopeless of execution, was in itself a good one, and that men, though excused from lighter labors, ought to take an equal share in the severer,— adding, that she wished the missionaries would give their husbands medicine and make them work.

The health of educated womanhood in the different European nations seems to depend mainly upon the degree of conformity to these rustic habits of air and exercise. In Italy, Spain, Portugal, the women of the upper classes lead secluded and unhealthy lives, and hence their physical condition is not superior to our own. In the Northern nations, women of refinement do more to emulate the active habits of the peasantry, — only substituting out-door relaxations for out-door toil, — and so they share their health. This is especially the case in England, which accordingly seems to furnish the representative types of vigorous womanhood. "The nervous system of the female sex in England seems to be of a much stronger mould than that of other nations," says Dr. Merei, a medical practitioner of English and Continental experience. "They bear a degree of irritation in their systems, without the issue of fits, which in other races is not so easily tolerated." So Professor Tyndall, watching female pedestrianism among the Alps, exults in his countrywomen: "The contrast in regard to energy between the maidens of the British Isles and those of the Continent and of America is astonishing." When Catlin's Indians first walked the streets of London, they reported with wonder that they had seen many handsome squaws holding to the arms of men, "and they did not look sick either"; — a remark which no complimentary savage was ever heard to make in any Cisatlantic metropolis.

There is undoubtedly an impression in this country that the English vigor is bought at some sacrifice, — that it implies a nervous organization less fine and artistic, features and limbs more rudely moulded, and something more coarse and peasant-like in the whole average texture. Making all due allowance for national vanity, it is yet easy to see that superiority may be had more cheaply by lowering the plane of attainment. The *physique* of a healthy day-laborer is a thing of inferior mould to the *physique* of a healthy artist. Muscular power needs also nervous power to bring out its finest quality. Lightness and grace are not incompatible with vigor, but are its crowning illustration. Apollo is above Hercules; Hebe and Diana are winged, not weighty. The physiologist must never forget that Nature is aiming at a keener and subtiler temperament in framing the American, — as beneath our drier atmosphere the whole scale of sounds and hues and odors is tuned to a higher key, — and that for us an equal state of health may yet produce a higher type of humanity. To make up the arrears of past neglect, therefore, is a matter of absolute necessity, if we wish this experiment of national temperament to have any chance; since rude health, however obtuse, will in the end overmatch disease, however finely strung.

But the fact must always be kept in mind, that the whole problem of female health is most closely intertwined with that of social conditions. The Anglo-Saxon organization is being modified not only in America, but also in England, with the changing habits of the people. In the days of Henry VIII. it was "a wyve's occupation to winnow all manner of cornes, to make malte, to wash and ironyng, to make hay, shere corne, and in time of nede to help her husband fill the muchpayne, drive the plough, load hay, corne, and such other, and go or ride to the market to sell butter, cheese, egges, chekyns, capons, hens, pigs, geese, and all manner of cornes." But now there is everywhere complaint of the growing delicacy and fragility of the English female population, even in rural regions; and the king of sanitary reformers, Edwin

Chadwick, has lately made this complaint the subject of a special report before the National Association. He assumes, as a matter settled by medical authority, that the proportion of mothers who can suckle their children is decidedly diminishing among the upper and middle classes, that deaths from childbirth are eight times as great among these classes as among the peasantry, and that spinal distortion, hysteria, and painful disorders are on the increase. Nine tenths of the evil he attributes to the long hours of school study, and to the neglect of physical exercises for girls.

This shows that the symptoms of ill-health among women are not a matter of climate only, but indicate a change in social conditions, producing a change of personal habits. It is something which reaches all; for the standard of health in the farm-houses is with us no higher than in the cities. It is something which, unless removed, stands as a bar to any substantial progress in civilization. It is a mere mockery for the millionnaire to create galleries of Art, bringing from Italy a Venus on canvas or a stone Diana, if meanwhile a lovelier bloom than ever artist painted is fading from his own child's cheek, and a firmer vigor than that of marble is vanishing from her enfeebled arms. What use to found colleges for girls whom even the high-school breaks down, or to induct them into new industrial pursuits when they have not strength to stand behind a counter? How appeal to any woman to enlarge her thoughts beyond the mere drudgery of the household, when she "dies daily" beneath the exhaustion of even that?

And the perplexity lies beyond the disease, in the perils involved even in the remedy. No person can be long conversant with physical training, without learning to shrink from the responsibility of the health of girls. The panacea for boyish health is commonly simple, even in delicate cases. Removal from books, if necessary, and the substitution of farm-life, — with good food, pure air, dogs, horses, oxen, hens, rabbits, — and fresh or salt water within walking distance. Secure these conditions, and then let him alone; he will not hurt himself. Nor will, during mere childhood, his little sister experience anything but benefit, under the same circumstances. But at the epoch of womanhood, precisely when the constitution should be acquiring robust strength, her perils begin; she then needs not merely to be allured to exertion, but to be protected against over-exertion; experience shows that she cannot be turned loose, cannot be safely left with boyish freedom to take her fill of running, rowing, riding, swimming, skating, — because life-long injury may be the penalty of a single excess. This necessity for caution cannot be the normal condition, for such caution cannot be exerted for the female peasant or savage, but it seems the necessary condition for American young women. It is a fact not to be ignored, that some of the strongest and most athletic girls among us have lost their health and become invalids for years, simply by being allowed to live the robust, careless, indiscreet life on which boys thrive so wonderfully. It is fatal, if they do too little, and disastrous, if they do too much; and between these two opposing perils the process of steering is so difficult, that the majority of parents end in letting go the helm and leaving the fragile vessel to steer itself.

Everything that follows in these pages must therefore be construed in the light of this admitted difficulty. The health of boys is a matter not hard to treat, on purely physiological grounds; but in dealing with that of girls caution is necessary. Yet, after all, the perplexities can only obscure the details of the prescription, while the main substance is unquestionable. Nowhere in the universe, save in improved habits, can we ever find health for our girls. Special delicacy in the conditions of the problem only implies more sedulous care in the solution. The great laws of exercise, of respiration, of digestion, are essentially the same for all human beings; and greater sensitiveness in the patient should not relax, but only stimulate, our efforts after cure. And the unquestionable fact that there are among us, after the worst is said, large numbers of robust and healthy women, should keep up our courage until we can apply their standard to the whole sex.

In presence of an evil so great, it is inevitable that there should be some fantastic theories of cure. But extremes are quite pardonable, where it is so important to explore all the sources of danger. Special ills should have special assailants, at whatever risk of exaggeration. As water-cures and vegetarian boarding-houses are the necessary defence of humanity against dirt and over-eating, so is the most ungainly Bloomer that ever drifted on bare poles across the continent a providential protest against the fashion-plates. It is probable, that, on the whole, there is a gradual amelioration in female costume. These hooded water-proof cloaks, equalizing all womankind, — these thick soles and heavy heels, proclaiming themselves with such masculine emphasis on the pavement, — these priceless india-rubber boots, emancipating all juvenile femineity from the terrors of mud and snow,— all these indicate an approaching era of good sense; for they are the requisite machinery of air, exercise, and health, so far as they go.

The weight of skirts and the constraints of corsets are still properly made the theme of indignant declamation. Yet let us be just. It is impossible to make costume the prime culprit, when we recall what robust generations have been reared beneath the same formidable panoply. For instance, it seems as if no woman could habitually walk uninjured with a weight of twelve pounds of skirts suspended at her hips, — Dr. Coale is responsible for the statistics, — and as if salvation must therefore lie in shoulder-straps. Yet the practice cannot be sheer suicide, when the Dutch peasant-girl plods bloomingly through her daily duties beneath a dozen successive involucres of flannel. So in regard to tight lacing, no one can doubt its ill effects, since even a man's loose garments are known to diminish by one fourth his capacity for respiration. Yet inspect in the shop-windows (where the facts of female costume are obtruded too pertinaciously for the public to remain in ignorance) the light and flexible corsets of these days, and then contemplate at Pilgrim Hall in Plymouth the stout buckram stays that once incased the stouter heart of Alice Bradford. Those, again, were to those of a still earlier epoch as leather to chain-armor. The Countess of Buchan was confined in an iron cage for life for assisting to crown Robert the Bruce, but her only loss by the incarceration was that her iron cage ceased to be portable.

Passing from costume, it must be noticed that there are many physical evils which the American woman shares with the other sex, but which bear with far greater severity on her finer organization. There is improper food, for instance. The fried or salted meat, the heavy bread, the perennial pork, the disastrous mince-pies of our farmers' houses, are sometimes pardoned by Nature to the men of the family, in consideration of twelve or more hours of out-door labor. For the more sedentary and delicate daughter there is no such atonement, and she vibrates between dyspepsia and starvation. The only locality in America where I have ever found the farming population living habitually on wholesome diet is the Quaker region in Eastern Pennsylvania, and I have never seen anywhere else such a healthy race of women. Yet here, again, it is not safe to be hasty, or to lay the whole responsibility upon the kitchen, when we recall the astounding diet on which healthy Englishwomen subsisted two centuries ago. Consider, for instance, the housekeeping of the Duke of Northumberland. "My lord and lady have for breakfast, at seven o'clock, a quart of beer, as much wine, two pieces of salt fish, six red herring, four white ones, and a dish of sprats." Digestive resources which could entertain this bill of fare might safely be trusted to travel in America.

The educational excesses of our schools, also, though shared by both sexes, tell much more formidably upon girls, in proportion as they are keener students, more submissive pupils, and are given to studying their lessons at recess-time, instead of shouting and racing in the open air. They are also easily coerced into devoting Wednesday and Saturday afternoons to the added atrocity of music-lessons, and in general, but for the recent blessed innovation of skating, would undoubtedly submit to having every atom of air and exercise eliminated from their lives. It is rare to find an American mother who habitually ranks physical vigor first, in rearing her daughters, and intellectual culture only second; indeed, they are commonly satisfied with a merely negative condition of health. The girl is considered to be well, if she is not too ill to go to school; and she therefore lives from hand to mouth, as respects her constitution, and lays up nothing for emergencies. From this negative condition proceeds her inability to endure accidents which to an active boy would be trivial. Who ever hears of a boy's incurring a lame knee for a year by slipping on the ice, or spinal disease for a lifetime by a fall from a sled? And if a girl has not enough of surplus vitality to overcome such trifles as these, how is she fitted to meet the coming fatigues of wife and mother?

These are important, if superficial, suggestions; but there are other considerations which go deeper. I take the special provocatives of disease among American women to be in great part social. The one marked step achieved thus far by our civilization appears to be the abolition of the peasant class, among the native-born, and the elevation of the mass of women to the social zone of music-lessons and silk gowns. This implies the disappearance of field-labor for women, and, unfortunately, of that rustic health also which in other countries is a standing exemplar for all classes. Wherever the majority of women work in the fields, the privileged minority are constantly reminded that they also hold their health by the tenure of some substituted activity. With us, all women have been relieved from out-door labor, — and are being sacrificed in the process, until they learn to supply its place. Except the graceful and vanishing pursuit of hop-picking, there is in New England no agricultural labor in which women can be said to be habitually engaged. Most persons never saw an American woman making hay, unless in the highly imaginative cantata of "The Hay-Makers"; and Dolly the Dairy-Maid is becoming to our children as purely ideal a being as Cinderella. We thus lose not only the immediate effect, but the indirect example, of these out-door toils.

This influence of the social transition bears upon all women: there is another which especially touches wives and mothers. In European countries, the aim at anything like gentility implies keeping one or more domestics to perform household labors; but in our Free States every family aims at gentility, while not one in five keeps a domestic. The aim is not a foolish one, though follies may accompany it, — for the average ambition of our people includes a certain amount of refined cultivation; — it is only that the process is exhausting. Every woman must have a best-parlor with hair-cloth furniture and a photograph-book; she must have a piano, or some cheaper substitute; her little girls must have embroidered skirts and much mathematical knowledge; her husband must have two, or even three, hot meals every day of his life; and yet her house must be in perfect order early in the afternoon, and she prepared to go out and pay calls, with a black-silk dress and a card-case. In the evening she will go to a concert or a lecture, and then, at the end of all, she will very possibly sit up after midnight with her sewing-machine, doing extra shop-work to pay for little Ella's music-lessons. All this every "capable" New-England woman will do, or die. She does it, and dies; and then we are astonished that her vital energy gives out sooner than that of an Irishwoman in a shanty, with no ambition on earth but to supply her young Patricks with adequate potatoes.

Now it is useless to attempt to set back the great social flood. The New-England housekeeper will never be killed by idleness, at any rate; and if she is exposed to the opposite danger, we must fit her for it, that is all. There is reason to be hopeful; the human race as a whole is tending upward, even physically, and if we cannot make our girls healthy quite yet, we shall learn to do it by and by. Meanwhile we must hold hard to the conviction, that not merely decent health, but even a high physical training, is a thing thoroughly practicable for both sexes. If a young girl can tire out her partner in the dance, if a delicate wife can carry her baby twice as long as her athletic husband, (for certainly there is nothing in the gymnasium more amazing than the mother's left arm,) then it is evident that the female frame contains muscular power, or its equivalent, though it may take music or maternity to bring it out. But other inducements have proved sufficient, and the results do not admit of question. The Oriental *bayadères*, for instance, are trained from childhood as gymnasts: they carry heavy jars on their heads, to improve strength, gait, and figure; they fly kites, to acquire "statuesque attitudes and graceful surprises"; they must learn to lay the back of the hand flat against the wrist, to partially bend the arm in both directions at the elbow, and, inclining the whole person backward from the waist, to sweep the floor with the hair. So, among ourselves, the great athletic resources of the female frame are vindicated by every equestrian goddess of the circus, every pet of the ballet. Those airy nymphs have been educated for their vocation by an amount of physical fatigue which their dandy admirers may well prefer to contemplate through the safe remoteness of an opera-glass. Dr. Gardner, of New York, has lately contributed very important professional observations upon this class of his patients; he describes their *physique* as infinitely superior to that of ordinary women, wonderfully adapting them, not only to the extraordinary, but to the common perils of their sex, "with that happy union of power and pliability most to be desired." "Their occupation demands in its daily study and subsequent practice an amount of long-continued muscular energy of the severest character, little recognized or understood by the community"; and his description of their habitual immunity in the ordeals of womanhood reminds one of the descriptions of savage tribes. But it is really a singular retribution for our prolonged offences against the body, when our saints are thus compelled to take their models from the reputed sinners, — prize-fighters being propounded as missionaries for the men, and opera-dancers for the women.

Are we literally to infer, then, that dancing must be the primary prescription? It would not be a bad one. It was an invaluable hint of Hippocrates, that the second-best remedy is better than the best, if the patient likes it best. Beyond all other merits of the remedy in question is this crowning advantage, that the patient likes it. Has any form of exercise ever yet been invented which a young girl would not leave for dancing? "Women, it is well known," says Jean Paul, "cannot run, but only dance, and every one could more easily reach a given point by dancing than by walking." It is practised in this country under immense disadvantages: first, because of late hours and heated rooms; and secondly, because some of the current dances seem equally questionable to the mamma and the physiologist. But it is doubtful whether any possible gymnastic arrangement for a high-school would be on the whole so provocative of wholesome exercise as a special hall for dancing, thoroughly ventilated, and provided with piano and spring-floor. The spontaneous festivals of every recess-time would then rival those German public-rooms, where it is said you may see a whole company waltzing like teetotums, with the windows wide open, at four o'clock in the afternoon.

Skating is dancing in another form; both aim at flying, and skating comes nearest to success. The triumph of this art has been so astonishing, in the universality of its introduction among our girls within the short space of four winters, that it is hardly necessary to speak of it, except to deduce the hope that other out-door enjoyments, equally within the reach of girls, may be as easily popularized.

For any form of locomotion less winged than skating and dancing, the feet of American girls have hitherto seemed somehow unfitted by Nature. There is every abstract reason why they should love walking, on this side the Atlantic: there is plenty of room for it, the continent is large; the exercise, moreover, brightens the eye and purifies the complexion, — so the physiologists declare; so that an English chemist classifies red cheeks as being merely oxygen in another form, and advises young ladies who wish for a pair to seek them where the roses get them, out of doors, — upon which an impertinent damsel writes to ask "Punch" if they might not as well carry the imitation of the roses a little farther, and remain in their beds all the time? But it is a lamentable fact, that walking, for the mere love of it, is a rare habit among our young women, and rarer probably in the country than in the city; it is uncommon to hear of one who walks habitually as much as two miles a day. There are, of course, many exceptional instances: I know maidens who love steep paths and mountain rains, like Wordsworth's Louisa, and I have even heard of eight young ladies who walked from Andover to Boston, twenty-three miles, in six hours, and of two in Ohio who did forty-five miles in two days. Moreover, with our impulsive temperaments, a special object will always operate as a strong allurement. A confectioner's shop, for instance. A camp somewhere in the suburbs, with dress-parades, and available lieutenants. A new article of dress: a real ermine cape may be counted as good for three miles a day, for the season. A dearest friend within pedestrian distance: so that it would seem well to plant a circle of delightful families just in the outskirts of every town, merely to serve as magnets. Indeed, so desperate has the emergency become, that one might take even ladies' hoops to be a secret device of Nature to secure more exercise for the occupants by compelling them thus to make the circuit of each other, as the two fat noblemen at the French court vindicated themselves from the charge of indolence by declaring that each promenaded twice round his friend every morning.

In view of this distaste for pedestrian exercise, it seems strange that the present revival of athletic exercises has not yet reached to horsemanship, the traditional type of all noble training, *chevalerie*, chivalry. Certainly it is not for the want of horse-flesh, for never perhaps was so much of that costly commodity owned in this community; yet in New England you shall find private individuals who keep a half-dozen horses each, and livery-stables possessing fifty, and never a proper saddle-horse among them. In some countries, riding does half the work of physical training, for both sexes; Sir Walter Scott, when at Abbotsford, never omitted his daily ride, and took his little daughter with him, from the time she could sit on horseback; but what New-England man, in purchasing a steed, selects with a view to a side-saddle? This seems a sad result of the wheel-maker's trade, and one grudges

St. Willegis the wheel on his coat-of-arms, if it has thus served to tame down freeborn men and women to the slouching and indolent practice of driving, — a practice in which the human figure appears at such disadvantage, that one can hardly wonder at Horace Walpole's coachman, who had laid up a small fortune by driving the maids-of-honor, and left it all to his son upon condition that he never should take a maid-of-honor for his wife.

An exercise to which girls take almost as naturally as to dancing is that of rowing, an accomplishment thoroughly feminine, learned with great facility, and on the whole safer than most other sports. Yet until within a few years no one thought of it in connection with women, unless with semi-mythical beings, like Ellen Douglas or Grace Darling. Even now it is chiefly a city accomplishment, and you rarely find at rural or sea-side places a village damsel who has ever handled an oar. But once having acquired the art, girls will readily fatigue themselves with its practice, unsolicited, careless of tan and freckles. At Dove Harbor it is far easier at any time to induce the young ladies to row for two hours, than to walk in the beautiful wood-paths for fifteen minutes; — the walking tires them. No matter; for a special exercise the rowing is the most valuable of the two, and furnishes just what the dancing-school omits. Unfortunately, the element of water is not quite a universal possession, and no one can train Naiads on dry land.

One of the merits of boating is that it suggests indirectly the attendant accomplishment of swimming, and this is something of such priceless importance that no trouble can be too great for its acquisition. Parents are uneasy until their children are vaccinated, and yet leave them to incur a risk as great and almost as easily averted.

The barbarian mother, who, lowering her baby into the water by her girdle, teaches it to swim ere it can walk, is before us in this duty. Swimming, moreover, is not one of those arts in which a little learning is a dangerous thing; on the contrary, a little may be as useful in an emergency as a great deal, if it gives those few moments of self-possession amid danger which will commonly keep a person from drowning until assistance comes. Women are naturally as well fitted for swimming as men, since specific buoyancy is here more than a match for strength; but effort is often needed to secure for them those opportunities of instruction and practice which the unrestrained wanderings of boys secure for them so easily. For this purpose, swimming-schools for ladies are now established in many places, at home and abroad; and the newspapers have lately chronicled a swimming-match at a girl's school in Berlin, where thirty-three competitors were entered for the prize, — and another among titled ladies in Paris, where each fashionable swimmer was allowed the use of the left hand only, the right hand sustaining an open parasol. Our own waters have, it may be, exhibited spectacles as graceful, though less known to fame. Never may I forget the bevy of bright maidens who under my pilotage buffeted on many a summer's day the surges of Cape Ann, learning a wholly new delight in trusting the buoyancy of the kind old ocean and the vigor of their own fair arms. Ah, my pupils, some of you have since been a prince's partners in the ball-room; but in those days, among the dancing waves, it was King Neptune who placed on you his crown.

Other out-door habits depend upon the personal tastes of the individual, in certain directions, and are best cultivated by educating these. If a young girl is born and bred with a love of any branch of natural history or of horticulture, happy is she; for the mere unconscious interest of the pursuit is an added lease of life to her. It is the same with all branches of Art whose pursuit leads into the open air. Rosa Bonheur, with her wanderings among mountains and pastures, alternating with the vigorous work of the studio, needed no other appliances for health. The same advantages come to many, in spite of delinquent mothers, in the bracing habits of household labor, at least where mechanical improvements have not rendered it too easy. Improved cooking-stoves and Mrs. Cornelius have made the culinary art such a path of roses that it is hardly now included in early training, but deferred till after matrimony. Yet bread-making in well-ventilated kitchens and sweeping in open-windowed rooms are calisthenics so bracing that one grudges them to the Irish maidens, whose round and comely arms betray so much less need of their tonic influence than the shrunken muscles exhibited so freely by our short-sleeved belles.

Perhaps even well-developed arms are not so essential to female beauty as erectness of figure, a trait on which our low school-desks have made sad havoc. The only sure panacea for round shoulders in boys appears to be the military drill, and Miss Mitford records that in her youth it was the custom in girls' schools to apply the same remedy. Dr. Lewis relies greatly on the carrying of moderate weights upon a padded wooden cap which he has devised for this purpose; and certainly the straightest female figure with which I am acquainted — aged seventy-four — is said to have been formed by the youthful habit of pacing the floor for half an hour daily, with a book upon the head, under rigid maternal discipline. Another traditional method is to insist that the damsel shall sit erect, without leaning against the chair, for a certain number of hours daily; and Sir Walter Scott says that his mother, in her eightieth year, took as much care to avoid giving any support to her back as if she had been still under the stern eye of Mrs. Ogilvie, her early teacher. Such simple methods may not be enough to check diseased curvatures or inequalities when already formed: these are best met by Ling's system of medical gymnastics, or "movement-cure," as applied by Dr. Lewis, Dr. Taylor, and others.

The ordinary gymnastic apparatus has also been employed extensively by women, and that very successfully, wherever the exercises have been systematically organized, with agreeable classes and competent teachers. If the gymnasium often fails to interest girls as much as boys, it is probably from deficiency in these respects, — and also because the female pupils, beginning on a lower plane of strength, do not command so great a variety of exercises, and so tire of the affair more readily. But hundreds, if not thousands, of American women have practised in these institutions during the last ten years, — single establishments in large cities having sometimes several hundred pupils, — and many have attained a high degree of skill in climbing, vaulting, swinging, and the like; nor can I find that any undue proportion of accidents has occurred. Wherever Dr. Lewis's methods have been introduced, important advantages have followed. He has invented an astonishing variety of games and well-studied movements, — with the lightest and cheapest apparatus, balls, bags, rings, wands, wooden dumb-bells, small clubs, and other instrumentalities, — which are all gracefully and effectually used by his classes, to the sound of music, and in a way to spare the weakest when lightly administered, or to fatigue the strongest when applied in force. Being adapted for united use by both sexes, they make more thorough appeal to the social element than the ordinary gymnastics; and evening classes, to meet several evenings in a week, have proved exceedingly popular in some of our towns. These exercises do not require fixed apparatus or a special hall. For this and other reasons they are peculiarly adapted for use in schools, and it would be well if they could be regularly taught in our normal institutions. Dr. Lewis himself is now training regular teachers to carry on the same good work, and his movement is undoubtedly the most important single step yet taken for the physical education of American women.

There is withal a variety of agreeable minor exercises, dating back farther than gymnastic professors, which must not be omitted. Archery, still in fashion in England, has never fairly taken root among us, and seems almost hopeless: the clubs formed for its promotion die out almost as speedily as cricket-clubs, and leave no trace behind; though this may not always be. Bowling and billiards are, however, practised by lady amateurs, just so far as they find opportunity, which is not very far; desirable public or private facilities being obtainable by few only, except at the summer watering-places. Battledoor-and-shuttlecock seems likely to come again into favor, and that under eminent auspices: Dr. Windship holding it in high esteem, as occupying the mind while employing every part of the body, harmonizing the muscular system, giving quickness to eye and hand, and improving the balancing power. The English, who systematize all amusements so much more than we, have developed this simple entertainment into several different games, arduous and complicated as their games of ball. The mere multiplication of the missiles also lends an additional stimulus, and the statistics of success in this way appear almost fabulous. A zealous English battledoorean informs me that the highest sçores yet recorded in the game are as follows: five thousand strokes for a single shuttlecock, five hundred when employing two, one hundred and fifty with three, and fifty-two when four airy messengers are kept flying simultaneously.

It may seem trivial to urge upon rational beings the use of a shuttlecock as a duty; but this is surely better than that one's health should become a thing as perishable, and fly away as easily. There is no danger that our educational systems will soon grow too careless of intellect and too careful of health. Reforms, whether in physiology or in smaller things, move slowly, when prejudice or habit bars the way. Paris is the head-quarters of medical science; yet in Paris, to this day, the poor babies in the great hospital of La Maternité are so tortured in tight swathings that not a limb can move. Progress is not in proportion to the amount of scientific knowledge on deposit in any country, but to the extent of its diffusion. No nation in the world grapples with its own evils so promptly as ours. It is but a few years since there was a general croaking about the physical deterioration of young men in our cities, — and now already the cities and the colleges are beginning to lead the rural districts in this respect. The guaranty of reform in American female health is to be found in the growing popular conviction that reform is needed. The community is tired of the reproaches of foreigners, and of the more serious evils of homes desolated by disease, and lives turned to tragedies. Morbid anatomy has long enough served as a type of feminine loveliness; our polite society has long enough been a series of *soirées* of incurables. Health is coming into fashion. A mercantile parent lately told me that already in his town, if a girl could vault a five-barred gate, her prospects for a husband were considered to be improved ten per cent; and every one knows that there is no meter of public sentiment so infallible as the stock-market. Now that the country is becoming safe, we must again turn our attention to the health of our girls. Unless they are healthy, the country is not safe. Nowhere can their physical condition be so important as in a republic. The utmost attention was paid to the bodily training of Victoria, because she was to be a queen and the mother of kings. By the theory of our government, however imperfectly applied as yet, this is the precise position of every American girl. Voltaire said that the fate of nations had often depended on the gout of a prime-minister; and the fate of our institutions may hang on the precise temperament which our next President shall have inherited from his mother.

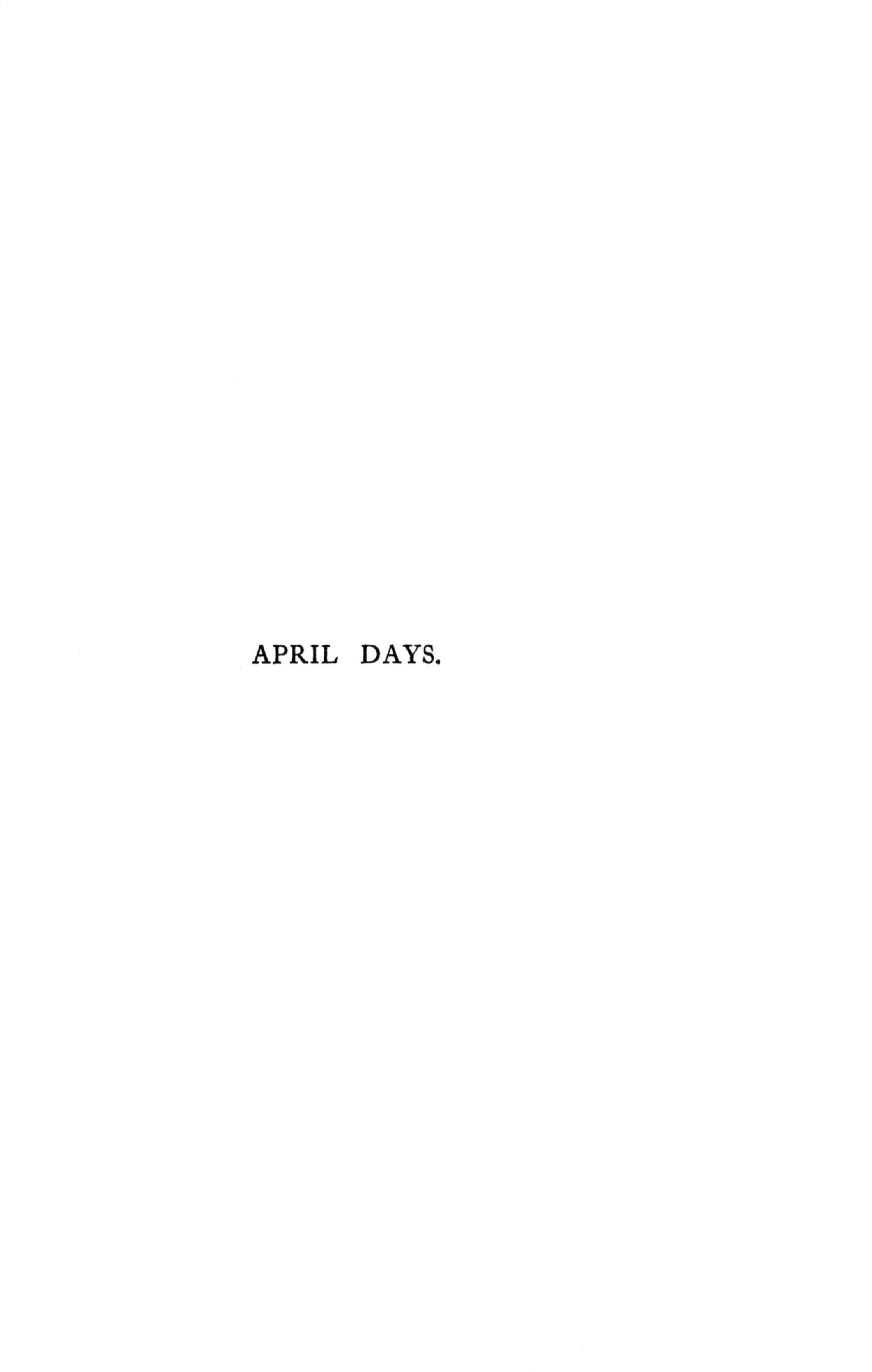

APRIL DAYS.

APRIL DAYS.

> "Can trouble dwell with April days?"
>
> *In Memoriam.*

IN our methodical New-England life, we still recognize some magic in summer. Most persons at least resign themselves to being decently happy in June. They accept June. They compliment its weather. They complain of the earlier months as cold, and so spend them in the city; and they complain of the later months as hot, and so refrigerate themselves on some barren sea-coast. God offers us yearly a necklace of twelve pearls; most men choose the fairest, label it June, and cast the rest away. It is time to chant a hymn of more liberal gratitude.

There are no days in the whole round year more delicious than those which often come to us in the latter half of April. On these days one goes forth in the morning, and finds an Italian warmth brooding over all the hills, taking visible shape in a glistening mist of silvered azure, with which mingles the smoke from many bonfires. The sun trembles in his own soft rays, till one understands the old English tradition, that he dances on Easter-Day. Swimming in a sea of glory, the tops of the hills look nearer than their bases, and their glistening watercourses seem close to the eye, as is their liberated murmur to the ear. All across this broad intervale the teams are ploughing. The grass in the meadow seems all to have grown green since yesterday. The blackbirds jangle in the oak, the robin is perched upon the elm, the song-sparrow on the hazel, and the bluebird on the apple-tree. There rises a hawk and sails slowly, the stateliest of airy things, a floating dream of long and languid summer-hours. But as yet, though there is warmth enough for a sense of luxury, there is coolness enough for exertion. No tropics can offer such a burst of joy; indeed, no zone much warmer than our Northern States can offer a genuine spring. There can be none where there is no winter, and the monotone of the seasons is broken only by wearisome rains. Vegetation and birds being distributed over the year, there is no burst of verdure nor of song. But with us, as the buds are swelling, the birds are arriving; they are building their nests almost simultaneously; and in all the Southern year there is no such rapture of beauty and of melody as here marks every morning from the last of April onward.

But days even earlier than these in April have a charm, — even days that seem raw and rainy, when the sky is dull and a bequest of March-wind lingers, chasing the squirrel from the tree and the children from the meadows. There is a fascination in walking through these bare early woods, — there is such a pause of preparation, winter's work is so cleanly and thoroughly done. Everything is taken down and put away; throughout the leafy arcades the branches show no remnant of last year, save a few twisted leaves of oak and beech, a few empty seed-vessels of the tardy witch-hazel, and a few gnawed nutshells dropped coquettishly by the squirrels into the crevices of the bark. All else is bare, but prophetic:

buds everywhere, the whole splendor of the coming summer concentrated in those hard little knobs on every bough; and clinging here and there among them, a brown, papery chrysalis, from which shall yet wave the superb wings of the Luna moth. An occasional shower patters on the dry leaves, but it does not silence the robin on the outskirts of the wood: indeed, he sings louder than ever during rain, though the song-sparrow and the bluebird are silent.

Then comes the sweetness of the nights in latter April. There is as yet no evening-primrose to open suddenly, no cistus to drop its petals; but the May-flower knows the hour, and becomes more fragrant in the darkness, so that one can then often find it in the woods without aid from the eye. The pleasant night-sounds are begun; the hylas are uttering their shrill *peep* from the meadows, mingled soon with hoarser toads, who take to the water at this season to deposit their spawn. The tree-toads soon join them; but one listens in vain for bullfrogs, or katydids, or grasshoppers, or whippoorwills, or crickets: we must wait for most of these until the delicious June.

The earliest familiar token of the coming season is the expansion of the stiff catkins of the alder into soft, drooping tresses. These are so sensitive, that, if you pluck them at almost any time during the winter, a few days' sunshine will make them open in a vase of water, and thus they eagerly yield to every moment of April warmth. The blossom of the birch is more delicate, that of the willow more showy, but the alders come first. They cluster and dance everywhere upon the bare boughs above the watercourses; the blackness of the buds is softened into rich brown and yellow; and as this graceful creature thus comes waving into the spring, it is pleasant to remember that the Norse Eddas fabled the first woman to have been named Embla, because she was created from an alder-bough.

The first wild-flower of the spring is like land after sea. The two which, throughout the Northern Atlantic States, divide this interest, are the *Epigæa repens* (May-flower, ground-laurel, or trailing-arbutus) and the *Hepatica triloba* (liverleaf, liverwort, or blue anemone). Of these two, the latter is perhaps more immediately exciting on first discovery; because it is an annual, not a perennial, — does not, like the epigæa, exhibit its buds all winter, but opens its blue eyes almost as soon as it emerges from the ground. Without the rich and delicious odor of its compeer, it has an inexpressibly fresh and earthy scent, that seems to bring all the promise of the blessed season with it; indeed, that clod of fresh turf with the inhalation of which Lord Bacon delighted to begin the day must undoubtedly have been full of the roots of our little hepatica. Its healthy sweetness belongs to the opening year, like Chaucer's poetry; and one thinks that anything more potent and voluptuous would be less enchanting — until one turns to the May-flower. Then comes a richer fascination for the senses. To pick the May-flower is like following in the footsteps of some spendthrift army which has scattered the contents of its treasure-chest among beds of scented moss. The fingers sink in the soft, moist verdure, and make at each instant some superb discovery unawares; again and again, straying carelessly, they clutch some new treasure; and, indeed, all is linked together in bright necklaces by secret threads beneath the surface, and where you grasp at one, you hold many. The hands go wandering over the moss as over the keys of a piano, and bring forth odors for melodies. The lovely creatures twine and nestle and lay their glowing faces to the very earth beneath withered leaves, and what seemed mere barrenness becomes fresh and fragrant beauty. So great is the charm of the pursuit, that the epigæa is really the wild-flower for which our country-people have a hearty passion. Every village child knows its best haunts, and watches for it eagerly in the spring; boys wreathe their hats with it, girls twine it in their hair, and the cottage-windows are filled with its beauty.

In collecting these early flowers, one finds or fancies singular natural affinities. I flatter myself with being able always to discover hepatica, if there is any within reach, for I was brought up with it ("Cockatoo he know me very well"); but other persons, who were brought up with May-flower, and remember searching for it with their almost baby-fingers, can find that better. The most remarkable instance of these natural affinities was in the case of L. T. and his double anemones. L. had always a gift for wild-flowers, and used often to bring to Cambridge the largest white anemones that ever were seen, from a certain special hill in Watertown; they were not only magnificent in size and whiteness, but had that exquisite blue on the outside of the petals, as if the sky had bent down in ecstasy at last over its darlings, and left visible kisses there. But even this success was not enough, and one day he came with something yet choicer. It was a rue-leaved anemone (*A. thalictroides*); and, if you will believe it, each one of the three white flowers was *double*, not merely with that multiplicity of petals in the disk which is common with this species, but technically and horticulturally double, like the double-flowering almond or cherry, — with the most exquisitely delicate little petals, like fairy lace-work. He had three specimens, —

gave one to the Autocrat of Botany, who said it was almost or quite unexampled, and another to me. As the man in the fable says of the chameleon, — "I have it yet, and can produce it."

Now comes the marvel. The next winter L. went to New York for a year, and wrote to me, as spring drew near, with solemn charge to visit his favorite haunt and find another specimen. Armed with this letter of introduction, I sought the spot, and tramped through and through its leafy corridors. Beautiful wood-anemones I found, to be sure, trembling on their fragile stems, deserving all their pretty names, — Wind-flower, Easter-flower, Pasque-flower, and homœopathic Pulsatilla; rue-leaved anemones I found also, rising taller and straighter and firmer in stem, with the whorl of leaves a little higher up on the stalk than one fancies it ought to be, as if there were a supposed danger that the flowers would lose their balance, and as if the leaves must be all ready to catch them. These I found, but the special wonder was not there for me. Then I wrote to L. that he must evidently come himself and search; or that, perhaps, as Sir Thomas Browne avers that "smoke doth follow the fairest," so his little treasures had followed him towards New York. Judge of my surprise, when, on opening his next letter, out dropped, from those folds of metropolitan paper, a veritable double anemone. He had just been out to Hoboken, or some such place, to spend an afternoon, and, of course, his pets were there to meet him; and from that day to this, I have never heard of the thing happening to any one else.

May-Day is never allowed to pass in this community without profuse lamentations over the tardiness of our spring as compared with that of England and the poets.

Yet it is easy to exaggerate this difference. Even so good an observer as Wilson Flagg is betrayed into saying that the epigæa and hepatica "seldom make their appearance until after the middle of April" in Massachusetts, and that "it is not unusual for the whole month of April to pass away without producing more than two or three species of wild-flowers." But I have formerly found the hepatica in bloom at Mount Auburn, for three successive years, on the twenty-seventh of March; and it has since been found in Worcester on the seventeenth, and in Danvers on the twelfth. The May-flower is usually as early, though the more gradual expansion of the buds renders it less easy to give dates. And there are nearly twenty species which I have noted, for five or six years together, as found always before May-Day, and which may therefore be properly assigned to April. The list includes bloodroot, cowslip, houstonia, saxifrage, dandelion, chickweed, cinquefoil, strawberry, mouse-ear, bellwort, dog's-tooth violet, five species of violet proper, and two of anemone. These are all common flowers, and easily observed; and the catalogue might be increased by rare ones, as the white corydalis, the smaller yellow violet (*V. rotundifolia*), and the claytonia or spring-beauty.

But in England the crocus and the snowdrop — neither being probably an indigenous flower, since neither is mentioned by Chaucer — usually open before the first of March; indeed, the snowdrop was formerly known by the yet more fanciful name of "Fair Maid of February." Chaucer's daisy comes equally early; and March brings daffodils, narcissi, violets, daisies, jonquils, hyacinths, and marsh-marigolds. This is altogether in advance of our season, so far as the wild-flowers give evidence, — though snowdrops are sometimes found in February even here.

But, on the other hand, it would appear that, though a larger number of birds winter in England than in Massachusetts, yet the return of those which migrate is actually earlier among us. From journals kept during sixty years in England, and an abstract of which is printed in Hone's "Every-Day Book," it appears that only two birds of passage revisit England before the fifteenth of April, and only thirteen more before the first of May; while with us the song-sparrow, the blue-bird, and the red-wing appear about the first of March, and quite a number more by the middle of April. This is a peculiarity of the English spring which I have never seen explained or even mentioned.

After the epigæa and the hepatica have opened, there is a slight pause among the wild-flowers, — these two forming a distinct prologue for their annual drama, as the brilliant witch-hazel in October brings up its separate epilogue. The truth is, Nature attitudinizes a little, liking to make a neat finish with everything, and then to begin again with *éclat.* Flowers seem spontaneous things enough, but there is evidently a secret marshalling among them, that all may be brought out with due effect. As the country-people say that so long as any snow is left on the ground more snow may be expected, it must all vanish simultaneously at last, — so every seeker of spring-flowers has observed how accurately they seem to move in platoons, with little straggling. Each species seems to burst upon us with a united impulse; you may search for them day after day in vain, but the day when you find one specimen the spell is broken and you find twenty. By the end of April all the margins of the great poem of the woods are illuminated with these exquisite vignettes.

Most of the early flowers either come before the full unfolding of their leaves, or else have inconspicuous ones. Yet Nature always provides for her bouquets the due proportion of green. The verdant and graceful sprays of the wild raspberry are unfolded very early, long before its time of flowering. Over the meadows spread the regular Chinese-pagodas of the equisetum (horsetail or scouring-rush), and the rich coarse vegetation of the veratrum, or American hellebore. In moist copses the ferns and osmundas begin to uncurl in April, opening their soft coils of spongy verdure, coated with woolly down, from which the humming-bird steals the lining of her nest.

The early blossoms represent the aboriginal epoch of our history: the bloodroot and the May-flower are older than the white man, older perchance than the red man; they alone are the true Native Americans. Of the later wild plants, many of the most common are foreign importations. In our sycophancy we attach grandeur to the name *exotic:* we call aristocratic garden-flowers by that epithet; yet they are no more exotic than the humbler companions they brought with them, which have become naturalized. The dandelion, the buttercup, chickweed, celandine, mullein, burdock, yarrow, whiteweed, nightshade, and most of the thistles, — these are importations. Miles Standish never crushed these with his heavy heel as he strode forth to give battle to the savages; they never kissed the daintier foot of Priscilla, the Puritan maiden. It is noticeable that these are all of rather coarser texture than our indigenous flowers; the children instinctively recognize this, and are apt to omit them, when gathering the more delicate native blossoms of the woods.

There is something touching in the gradual retirement before civilization of these fragile aborigines. They do not wait for the actual brute contact of red bricks and curbstones, but they feel the danger miles away. The Indians called the low plantain "the white man's footstep"; and these shy creatures gradually disappear, the moment the red man gets beyond their hearing. Bigelow's delightful "Florula Bostoniensis" is becoming a series of epitaphs. Too well we know it, — those of us who in happy Cambridge childhood often gathered, almost within a stone's throw of Professor Agassiz's new Museum, the arethusa and the gentian, the cardinal-flower and the gaudy rhexia, — we who remember the last secret hiding-place of the rhodora in West Cambridge, of the yellow violet and the *Viola debilis* in Watertown, of the *Convallaria trifolia* near Fresh Pond, of the *Hottonia* beyond Wellington's Hill, of the *Cornus florida* in West Roxbury, of the *Clintonia* and the dwarf ginseng in Brookline, — we who have found in its one chosen nook the sacred *Andromeda polyfolia* of Linnæus. Now vanished almost or wholly from city suburbs, these fragile creatures still linger in more rural parts of Massachusetts; but they are doomed everywhere, unconsciously, yet irresistibly; while others still more shy, as the *Linnæa*, the yellow *Cypripedium*, the early pink *Azalea*, and the delicate white *Corydalis* or "Dutchman's breeches," are being chased into the very recesses of the Green and the White Mountains. The relics of the Indian tribes are supported by the Legislature at Martha's Vineyard, while these precursors of the Indian are dying unfriended away.

And with these receding plants go also the special insects which haunt them. Who that knew that pure enthusiast, Dr. Harris, but remembers the accustomed lamentations of the entomologist over the departure of these winged companions of his lifetime? Not the benevolent Mr. John Beeson more tenderly mourns the decay of the Indians, than he the exodus of these more delicate native tribes. In a letter which I happened to receive from him a short time previous to his death, he thus renewed the lament: "I mourn for the loss of many of the beautiful plants and insects that were once found in this vicinity. *Clethra, Rhodora, Sanguinaria, Viola debilis, Viola acuta, Dracæna borealis, Rhexia, Cypripedium, Corallorhiza verna, Orchis spectabilis,* with others of less note, have been rooted out by the so-called hand of improvement. *Cicindela rugifrons, Helluo præusta, Sphæroderus stenostomus, Blethisa quadricollis* (*Americana mî*), *Carabus, Horia* (which for several years occurred in profusion on the sands beyond Mount Auburn), with others, have entirely disappeared from their former haunts, driven away, or exterminated perhaps, by the changes effected therein. There may still remain in your vicinity some sequestered spots, congenial to these and other rarities, which may reward the botanist and the entomologist who will search them carefully. Perhaps you may find there the pretty coccinella-shaped, silver-margined *Omophron*, or the still rarer *Panagæus fasciatus*, of which I once took two specimens on Wellington's Hill, but have not seen it since." Is not this indeed handling one's specimens "gently as if you loved them," as Isaak Walton bids the angler do with his worm?

There is this merit, at least, among the coarser crew of imported flowers, that they bring their own proper names with them, and we know precisely with whom we have to deal. In speaking of our own native flowers, we must either be careless and inaccurate, or else resort sometimes to the Latin, in spite of the indignation of friends. There is something yet to be said on this point. In England, where the old household and monkish names adhere, they are sufficient for popular and poetic purposes, and the familiar use of scientific names seems an affectation. But here, where many native flowers have no popular names at all, and others are called confessedly by wrong ones,— where it really costs less trouble to use Latin names than English,—the affectation seems the other way. Think of the long list of wild-flowers where the Latin name is spontaneously used by all who speak of the flower: as, Arethusa, Aster, Cistus ("after the fall of the cistus-flower"), Clematis, Clethra, Geranium, Iris, Lobelia, Rhodora, Spiræa, Tiarella, Trientalis, and so on. Even those formed from proper names (the worst possible system of nomenclature) become tolerable at last, and we forget the godfather in the more attractive namesake. Are those who pick the Houstonia to be supposed thereby to indorse the Texan President? Or are the deluded damsels who chew Cassia-buds to be regarded as swallowing the late Secretary of State? The names have long since been made over to the flowers, and every questionable aroma has vanished. When the person concerned happens to be a botanist, there is a peculiar fitness in the association; the Linnæa, at least, would not smell so sweet by any other name.

In other cases the English name is a mere modification of the Latin one, and our ideal associations have really a scientific basis: as with Violet, Lily, Laurel, Gentian, Vervain. Indeed, our enthusiasm for vernacular names is like that for Indian names of localities, one-sided: we enumerate only the graceful ones, and ignore the rest. It would be a pity to Latinize Touch-me-not, or Yarrow, or Gold-Thread, or Self-Heal, or Columbine, or Blue-Eyed-Grass, — though, to be sure, this last has an annoying way of shutting up its azure orbs the moment you gather it, and you reach home with a bare, stiff blade, which deserves no better name than *Sisyrinchium anceps.* But in what respect is Cucumber-Root preferable to Medeola, or Solomon's-Seal to Convallaria, or Rock-Tripe to Umbilicaria, or Lousewort to Pedicularis? In other cases the merit is divided: Anemone may dispute the prize of melody with Windflower, Campanula with Harebell, Neottia with Ladies'-Tresses, Uvularia with Bellwort and Strawbell, Potentilla with Cinquefoil, and Sanguinaria with Bloodroot. Hepatica may be bad, but Liverleaf is worse. The pretty name of May-flower is not so popular, after all, as that of Trailing-Arbutus, where the graceful and appropriate adjective redeems the substantive, which happens to be Latin and incorrect at the same time. It does seem a waste of time to say *Chrysanthemum leucanthemum* instead of Whiteweed; though, if the long scientific name were an incantation to banish the intruder, our farmers would gladly consent to adopt it.

But the great advantage of a reasonable use of the botanical name is, that it does not deceive us. Our primrose is not the English primrose, any more than it was our robin who tucked up the babes in the wood; our cowslip is not the English cowslip, it is the English marsh-marigold, — Tennyson's marsh-marigold. The pretty name of Azalea means something definite; but its rural name of Honeysuckle confounds under that name flowers without even an external resemblance, — Azalea, Diervilla, Lonicera, Aquilegia, — just as every bird which sings loud in deep woods is popularly denominated a thrush. The really rustic names of both plants and animals are very few with us, — the different species are many; and as we come to know them better and love them more, we absolutely require some way to distinguish them from their half-sisters and second-cousins. It is hopeless to try to create new popular epithets, or even to revive those which are thoroughly obsolete. Miss Cooper may strive in vain, with benevolent intent, to christen her favorite spring blossoms "May-Wings" and "Gay-Wings," and "Fringe-Cup" and "Squirrel-Cup," and "Cool-Wort" and "Bead-Ruby"; there is no conceivable reason why these should not be the familiar appellations, except the irresistible fact that they are not. It is impossible to create a popular name: one might as well attempt to invent a legend or compose a ballad. *Nascitur, non fit.*

As the spring comes on, and the densening outlines of the elm give daily a new design for a Grecian urn, — its hue first brown with blossoms, then emerald with leaves, — we appreciate the vanishing beauty of the bare boughs. In our favored temperate zone, the trees denude themselves each year, like the goddesses before Paris, that we may see which unadorned loveliness is the fairest. Only the unconquerable delicacy of the beech still keeps its soft vestments about it: far into spring, when worn to thin rags and tatters, they cling there still; and when they fall, the new appear as by magic. It must be owned, however, that the beech has good reasons for this prudishness, and possesses little beauty of figure; while the elms, maples, chestnuts, walnuts, and even oaks, have not exhausted all their store of charms for us, until we have seen them disrobed. Only yonder magnificent pine-tree, — that pitch-pine, nobler when seen in perfection than white-pine, or Norwegian, or Norfolk-Islander, — that pitch-pine, herself a grove, *una nemus*, holds her unchanging beauty throughout the year, like her half-brother, the ocean, whose voice she shares; and only marks the flowing of her annual tide of life by the new verdure that yearly submerges all trace of last year's ebb.

How many lessons of faith and beauty we should lose if there were no winter in our year! Sometimes in following up a watercourse among our hills, in the early spring, one comes to a weird and desolate place, where one huge wild grape-vine has wreathed its ragged arms around a whole thicket and brought it to the ground,—swarming to the tops of hemlocks, clenching a dozen young maples at once and tugging them downward, stretching its wizard black length across the underbrush, into the earth and out again, wrenching up great stones in its blind, aimless struggle. What a piece of chaos is this! Yet come here again, two months hence, and you shall find all this desolation clothed with beauty and with fragrance, one vast bower of soft green leaves and graceful tendrils, while summer birds chirp and flutter amid these sunny arches all the livelong day.

To the end of April, and often later, one still finds remains of snow-banks in sheltered woods, especially among evergreens; and this snow, like that upon high mountains, has often become hardened by the repeated thawing and freezing of the surface, till it is more impenetrable than ice. But the snow that falls during April is usually what Vermonters call "sugar-snow,"—falling in the night and just whitening the surface for an hour or two, and taking its name, not so much from its looks as from the fact that it denotes the proper weather for "sugaring," namely, cold nights and warm days. Our saccharine associations, however, remain so obstinately tropical, that it seems almost impossible for the imagination to locate sugar in New-England trees; though it is known that not the maple only, but the birch and the walnut even, afford it in appreciable quantities.

Along our maritime rivers the people associate April, not with "sugaring," but with "shadding." The pretty *Amelanchier Canadensis* of Gray — the *Aronia* of Whittier's song — is called Shad-bush or Shad-blow in Essex County, from its connection with this season; and there is a bird known as the Shad-spirit, which I take to be identical with the flicker or golden-winged woodpecker, whose note is still held to indicate the first day when the fish ascend the river. Upon such slender wings flits our New-England romance!

In April the creative process described by Thales is repeated, and the world is renewed by water. The submerged creatures first feel the touch of spring, and many an equivocal career, beginning in the ponds and brooks, learns later to ignore this obscure beginning, and hops or flutters in the dusty daylight. Early in March, before the first male canker-moth appears on the elm-tree, the whirlwig beetles have begun to play round the broken edges of the ice, and the caddis-worms to crawl beneath it; and soon come the water-skater (*Gerris*) and the water-boatman (*Notonecta*). Turtles and newts are in busy motion when the spring-birds are only just arriving. Those gelatinous masses in yonder wayside pond are the spawn of water-newts or tritons: in the clear transparent jelly are imbedded, at regular intervals, little blackish dots; these elongate rapidly, and show symptoms of head and tail curled up in a spherical cell; the jelly is gradually absorbed for their nourishment, until on some fine morning each elongated dot gives one vigorous wriggle, and claims thenceforward all the privileges attendant on this dissolution of the union. The final privilege is often that of being suddenly snapped up by a turtle or a snake: for Nature brings forth her creatures liberally, especially the aquatic ones, sacrifices nine tenths of them as food for their larger cousins, and reserves only a handful to propagate their race, on the same profuse scale, next season.

It is surprising, in the midst of our Museums and Scientific Schools, how little we yet know of the common things around us. Our *savans* still confess their inability to discriminate with certainty the egg or tadpole of a frog from that of a toad; and it is strange that these hopping creatures, which seem so unlike, should coincide so nearly in their juvenile career, while the tritons and salamanders, which border so closely on each other in their maturer state as sometimes to be hardly distinguishable, yet choose different methods and different elements for laying their eggs. The eggs of our salamanders or land-lizards are deposited beneath the moss on some damp rock, without any gelatinous envelope; they are but few in number, and the anxious mamma may sometimes be found coiled in a circle around them, like the symbolic serpent of eternity.

The small number of birds yet present in early April gives a better opportunity for careful study, — more especially if one goes armed with that best of fowling-pieces, a small spy-glass: the best, — since how valueless for purposes of observation is the bleeding, gasping, dying body, compared with the fresh and living creature, as it tilts, trembles, and warbles on the bough before you! Observe that robin in the oak-tree's top: as he sits and sings, every one of the dozen different notes which he flings down to you is accompanied by a separate flirt and flutter of his whole body, and, as Thoreau says of the squirrel, "each movement seems to imply a spectator." Study that song-sparrow: why is it that he always goes so ragged in spring, and the bluebird so neat? is it that the song-sparrow is a wild artist, absorbed in the composition of his lay, and oblivious of ordinary proprieties, while the smooth bluebird and his ash-colored mate cultivate their delicate warble only as a domestic accomplishment, and are always nicely dressed before sitting down to the piano? Then how exciting is the gradual arrival of the birds in their summer plumage! to watch it is as good as sitting at the window on Easter Sunday to observe the new bonnets. Yonder, in that clump of alders by the brook, is the delicious jargoning of the first flock of yellow-birds; there are the little gentlemen in black and yellow, and the little ladies in olive-brown; "sweet, sweet, sweet" is the only word they say, and often they will so lower their ceaseless warble, that, though almost within reach, the little minstrels seem far distant. There is the very earliest cat-bird, mimicking the bobolink before the bobolink has come: what is the history of his song, then? is it a reminiscence of last year? or has the little coquette been practising it all winter, in some gay Southern society, where cat-birds and bobolinks grow intimate, just as Southern fashionables from different States may meet and sing duets at Saratoga? There sounds the sweet, low, long-continued trill of the little hair-bird, or chipping-sparrow, a suggestion of insect sounds in sultry summer, and produced, like them, with the aid of a slight fluttering of the wings against the sides: by and by we shall sometimes hear that same delicate rhythm burst the silence of the June midnights, and then, ceasing, make stillness more still. Now watch that woodpecker, roving in ceaseless search, travelling over fifty trees in an hour, running from top to bottom of some small sycamore, pecking at every crevice, pausing to dot a dozen inexplicable holes in a row upon an apple-tree, but never once intermitting the low, querulous murmur of housekeeping anxiety: now she stops to hammer with all her little life at some tough piece of bark, strikes harder and harder blows, throws herself back at last, flapping her wings furiously as she brings down her whole strength again upon it; finally it yields, and grub after grub goes down her throat, till she whets her beak after the meal as a wild beast licks its claws, and off on her pressing business once more.

It is no wonder that there is so little substantial enjoyment of Nature in the community, when we feed children on grammars and dictionaries only, and take no pains to train them to see that which is before their eyes. The mass of the community have "summered and wintered" the universe pretty regularly, one would think, for a good many years; and yet nine persons out of ten in the town or city, and two out of three even in the country, seriously suppose, for instance, that the buds upon trees are formed in the spring; they have had them within sight all winter, and never seen them. So people suppose, in good faith, that a plant grows at the base of the stem, instead of at the top: that is, if they see a young sapling in which there is a crotch at five feet from the ground, they expect to see it ten feet from the ground by and by, — confounding the growth of a tree with that of a man or animal. But perhaps the best of us could hardly bear the system of tests unconsciously laid down by a small child of my acquaintance. The boy's father, a college-bred man, had early chosen the better part, and employed his fine faculties in rearing laurels in his own beautiful nursery-gardens, instead of in the more arid soil of court-rooms or state-houses. Of course the young human scion knew the flowers by name before he knew his letters, and used their symbols more readily; and after he got the command of both, he was one day asked by his younger brother what the word *idiot* meant, — for somebody in the parlor had been saying that somebody else was an idiot. "Don't you know?" quoth Ben, in his sweet voice: "an idiot is a person who does n't know an arbor-vitæ from a pine, — he does n't know anything." When Ben grows up to maturity, bearing such terrible definitions in his unshrinking hands, who of us will be safe?

The softer aspects of Nature, especially, require time and culture before man can enjoy them. To rude races her processes bring only terror, which is very slowly outgrown. Humboldt has best exhibited the scantiness of finer natural perceptions in Greek and Roman literature, in spite of the grand oceanic rhythm of Homer, and the delicate water-coloring of the Greek Anthology and of Horace. The Oriental and the Norse sacred books are full of fresh and beautiful allusions; but the Greek saw in Nature only a framework for Art, and the Roman only a camping-ground for men. Even Virgil describes the grotto of Æneas merely as a "black grove" with "horrid shade," — "*Horrenti atrum nemus imminet umbra.*" Wordsworth points out, that, even in English literature, the "Windsor Forest" of Anne, Countess of Winchelsea, was the first poem which represented Nature as a thing to be consciously enjoyed; and as she was almost the first English poetess, we might be tempted to think that we owe this appreciation, like some other good things, to the participation of woman in literature. But, on the other hand, it must be remembered that the voluminous Duchess of Newcastle, in her "Ode on Melancholy," describes among the symbols of hopeless gloom "the still moonshine night" and "a mill where rushing waters run about," — the sweetest natural images. So woman has not so much to claim, after all. In our own country, the early explorers seemed to find only horror in its woods and waterfalls. Josselyn, in 1672, could only describe the summer splendor of the White Mountain region as "dauntingly terrible, being full of rocky hills, as thick as molehills in a meadow, and full of infinite thick woods." Father Hennepin spoke of Niagara, in the narrative still quoted in the guide-books, as a "frightful cataract"; though perhaps his original French phrase was softer, and honest John Adams could find no better name than "horrid chasm" for the picturesque gulf at Egg Rock, where he first saw the sea-anemone.

But we are lingering too long, perhaps, with this sweet April of smiles and tears. It needs only to add, that all her traditions are beautiful. Ovid says well, that she was not named from *aperire*, to open, as some have thought, but from *Aphrodite*, goddess of beauty. April holds Easter-time, St. George's Day, and the Eve of St. Mark's. She has not, like her sister May in Germany, been transformed to a verb and made a synonyme for joy, — "*Deine Seele maiet den trüben Herbst*," — but April was believed in early ages to have been the birth-time of the world. According to Venerable Bede, the point was first accurately determined at a council held at Jerusalem about A. D. 200, when, after much profound discussion, it was finally decided that the world's birthday occurred on

Sunday, April 8th, — that is, at the vernal equinox and the full moon. But April is certainly the birth-time of the season, at least, if not of the planet. Its festivals are older than Christianity, older than the memory of man. No sad associations cling to it, as to the month of June, in which month, says William of Malmesbury, kings are wont to go to war, — "*Quando solent reges ad arma procedere*," — but it holds the Holy Week, and it is the Holy Month. And in April Shakespeare was born, and in April he died.

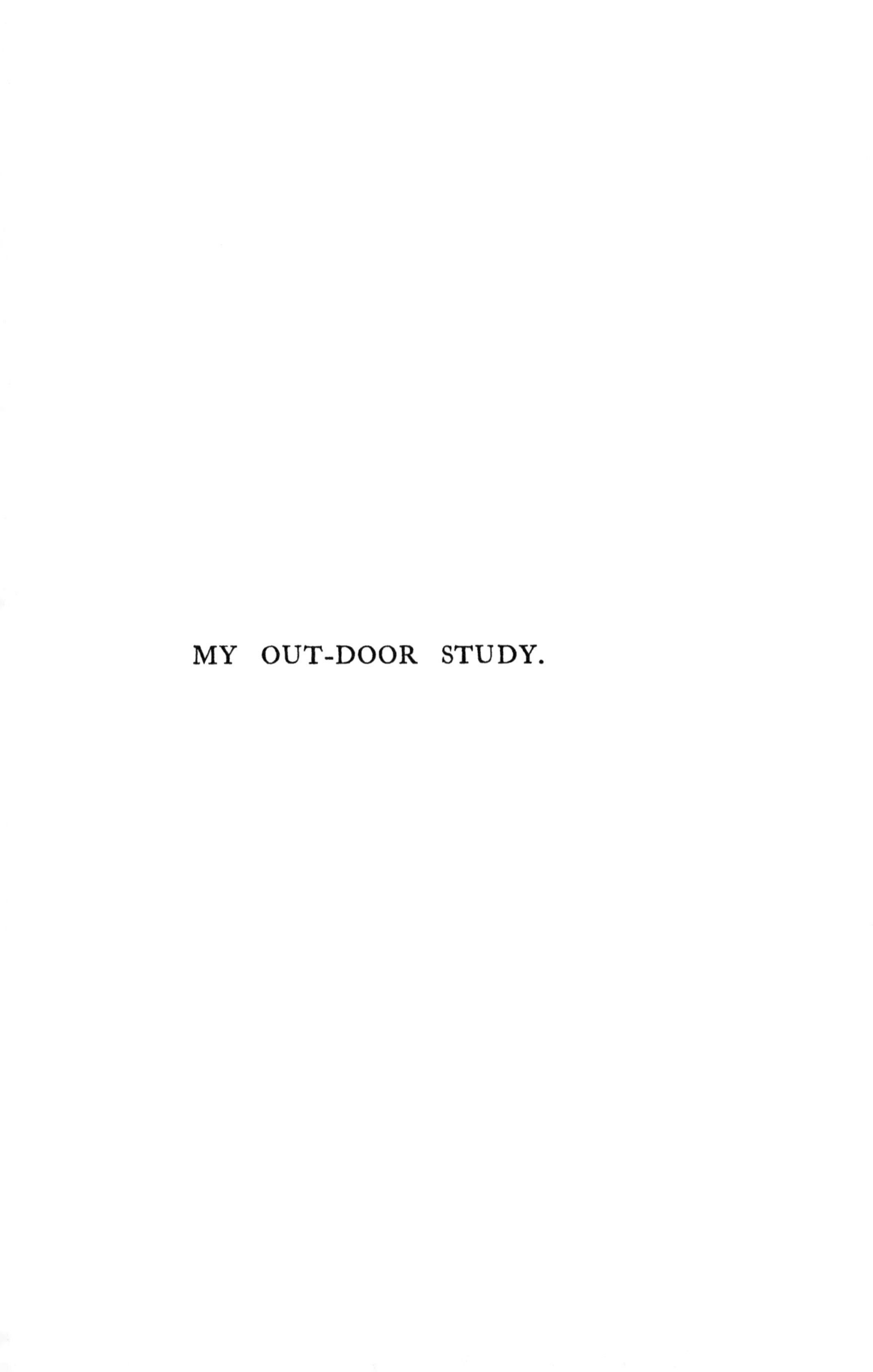

MY OUT-DOOR STUDY.

MY OUT-DOOR STUDY.

THE noontide of the summer day is past, when all Nature slumbers, and when the ancients feared to sing, lest the great god Pan should be awakened. Soft changes, the gradual shifting of every shadow on every leaf, begin to show the waning hours. Ineffectual thunder-storms have gathered and gone by, hopelessly defeated. The floating bridge is trembling and resounding beneath the pressure of one heavy wagon, and the quiet fishermen change their places to avoid the tiny ripple that glides stealthily to their feet above the half-submerged planks. Down the glimmering lake there are miles of silence and still waters and green shores, overhung with a multitudinous and scattered fleet of purple and golden clouds, now furling their idle sails and drifting away into the vast harbor of the South. Voices of birds, hushed first by noon and then by possibilities of tempest, cautiously begin once more, leading on the infinite melodies of the June afternoon. As the freshened air invites them forth, so the smooth and stainless water summons us. "Put your hand upon the oar," says Charon in the old play to Bacchus, "and you shall hear the sweetest songs." The doors of the boat-house swing softly open, and the slender wherry, like a water-snake, steals silently in the wake of the dispersing clouds.

The woods are hazy, as if the warm sunbeams had melted in among the interstices of the foliage and spread a soft film throughout the whole. The sky seems to reflect the water, and the water the sky; both are roseate with color, both are darkened with clouds, and between them both, as the boat recedes, the floating bridge hangs suspended, with its motionless fishermen and its moving team. The wooded islands are poised upon the lake, each belted with a paler tint of softer wave. The air seems fine and palpitating; the drop of an oar in a distant rowlock, the sound of a hammer on a dismantled boat, pass into some region of mist and shadows, and form a metronome for delicious dreams.

Every summer I launch my boat to seek some realm of enchantment beyond all the sordidness and sorrow of earth, and never yet did I fail to ripple with my prow at least the outskirts of those magic waters. What spell has fame or wealth to enrich this midday blessedness with a joy the more? Yonder barefoot boy, as he drifts silently in his punt beneath the drooping branches of yonder vine-clad bank, has a bliss which no Astor can buy with money, no Seward conquer with votes, — which yet is no monopoly of his, and to which time and experience only add a more subtile and conscious charm. The rich years were given us to increase, not to impair, these cheap felicities. Sad or sinful is the life of that man who finds not the heavens bluer and the waves more musical in maturity than in childhood. Time is a severe alembic of youthful joys, no doubt; we exhaust book after book, and leave Shakespeare unopened; we grow fastidious in men and women; all the rhetoric, all the logic, we fancy we have heard before; we have seen the pictures, we have listened to the symphonies: but what has been done by all the art and literature of the world towards describing one summer day? The most exhausting effort brings us no nearer to it than to the blue sky which is its dome; our words are shot up against it like arrows, and fall back helpless. Literary amateurs go the tour of the globe to renew their stock of materials, when they do not yet know a bird or a bee or a blossom beside their homestead-door; and in the hour of their greatest success they have not an horizon to their life so large as that of yon boy in his punt. All that is purchasable in the capitals of the world is not to be weighed in comparison with the simple enjoyment that may be crowded into one hour of sunshine. What can place or power do here? "Who could be before me, though the palace of Cæsar cracked and split with emperors, while I, sitting in silence on a cliff of Rhodes, watched the sun as he swung his golden censer athwart the heavens?"

It is pleasant to observe a sort of confused and latent recognition of all this in the instinctive sympathy which is always rendered to any indication of out-door pursuits. How cordially one sees the eyes of all travellers turn to the man who enters the railroad-station with a fowling-piece in hand, or the boy with water-lilies! There is a momentary sensation of the freedom of the woods, a whiff of oxygen for the anxious money-changers. How agreeably sounds the news — to all but his creditors — that the lawyer or the merchant has locked his office-door and gone fishing! The American temperament needs at this moment nothing so much as that wholesome training of semi-rural life which reared Hampden and Cromwell to assume at one grasp the sovereignty of England, and which has ever since served as the foundation of England's greatest ability. The best thoughts and purposes seemed ordained to come to human beings beneath the open sky, as the ancients fabled that Pan found the goddess Ceres when he was engaged in the chase, whom no other of the gods could find when seeking seriously. The little I have gained from colleges and libraries has certainly not worn so well as the little I learned in childhood of the habits of plant, bird, and insect. That "weight and sanity of thought," which Coleridge so finely makes the crowning attribute of Wordsworth, is in no way so well matured and cultivated as in the society of Nature.

There may be extremes and affectations, and Mary Lamb declared that Wordsworth held it doubtful if a dweller in towns had a soul to be saved. During the various phases of transcendental idealism among ourselves, in the last twenty years, the love of Nature has at times assumed an exaggerated and even a pathetic aspect, in the morbid attempts of youths and maidens to make it a substitute for vigorous thought and action, — a lion endeavoring to dine on grass and green leaves. In some cases this mental chlorosis reached such a height as almost to nauseate one with Nature, when in the society of the victims; and surfeited companions felt inclined to rush to the treadmill immediately, or get chosen on the Board of Selectmen, or plunge into any conceivable drudgery, in order to feel that there was still work enough in the universe to keep it sound and healthy. But this, after all, was exceptional and transitory, and our American life still needs, beyond all things else, the more habitual cultivation of out-door habits.

Probably the direct ethical influence of natural objects may be overrated. Nature is not didactic, but simply healthy. She helps everything to its legitimate development, but applies no goads, and forces on us no sharp distinctions. Her wonderful calmness, refreshing the whole soul, must aid both conscience and intellect in the end, but sometimes lulls both temporarily, when immediate issues are pending. The waterfall cheers and purifies infinitely, but it marks no moments, has no reproaches for indolence, forces to no immediate decision, offers unbounded to-morrows, and the man of action must tear himself away, when the time comes, since the work will not be done for him. "The natural day is very calm, and will hardly reprove our indolence."

And yet the more bent any man is upon action, the more profoundly he needs this very calmness of Nature to preserve his equilibrium. The radical himself needs nothing so much as fresh air. The world is called conservative; but it is far easier to impress a plausible thought on the complaisance of others, than to retain an unfaltering faith in it for ourselves. The most dogged reformer distrusts himself every little while, and says inwardly, like Luther, "Art thou alone wise?" So he is compelled to exaggerate, in the effort to hold his own. The community is bored by the conceit and egotism of the innovators; so it is by that of poets and artists, orators and statesmen; but if we knew how heavily ballasted all these poor fellows need to be, to keep an even keel amid so many conflicting tempests of blame and praise, we should hardly reproach them. But the simple enjoyments of out-door life, costing next to nothing, tend to equalize all vexations. What matter, if the Governor removes you from office? he cannot remove you from the lake; and if readers or customers will not bite, the pickerel will. We must keep busy, of course; yet we cannot transform the world except very slowly, and we can best preserve our patience in the society of Nature, who does her work almost as imperceptibly as we.

And for literary training, especially, the influence of natural beauty is simply priceless. Under the present educational systems, we need grammars and languages far less than a more thorough out-door experience. On this flowery bank, on this ripple-marked shore, are the true literary models. How many living authors have ever attained to writing a single page which could be for one moment compared, for the simplicity and grace of its structure, with this green spray of wild woodbine or yonder white wreath of blossoming clematis? A finely organized sentence should throb and palpitate like the most delicate vibrations of the summer air. We talk of literature as if it were a mere matter of rule and measurement, a series of processes long since brought to mechanical perfection: but it would be less incorrect to say that it all lies in the future; tried by the out-door standard, there is as yet no literature, but only glimpses and guideboards; no writer has yet succeeded in sustaining, through more than some single occasional sentence, that fresh and perfect charm. If by the training of a lifetime one could succeed in producing one continuous page of perfect cadence, it would be a life well spent, and such a literary artist would fall short of Nature's standard in quantity only, not in quality.

It is one sign of our weakness, also, that we commonly assume Nature to be a rather fragile and merely ornamental thing, and suited for a model of the graces only. But her seductive softness is the last climax of magnificent strength. The same mathematical law winds the leaves around the stem and the planets round the sun. The same law of crystallization rules the slight-knit snow-flake and the hard foundations of the earth. The thistle-down floats secure upon the same summer zephyrs that are woven into the tornado. The dew-drop holds within its transparent cell the same electric fire which charges the thunder-cloud. In the softest tree or the airiest waterfall, the fundamental lines are as lithe and muscular as the crouching haunches of a leopard; and without a pencil vigorous enough to render these, no mere mass of foam or foliage, however exquisitely finished, can tell the story. Lightness of touch is the crowning test of power.

Yet Nature does not work by single spasms only. That chestnut spray is not an isolated and exhaustive effort of creative beauty: look upward and see its sisters rise with pile above pile of fresh and stately verdure, till tree meets sky in a dome of glorious blossom, the whole as perfect as the parts, the least part as perfect as the whole. Studying the details, it seems as if Nature were a series of costly fragments with no coherency, — as if she would never encourage us to do anything systematically, — would tolerate no method but her own, and yet had none of her own, — were as abrupt in her transitions from oak to maple as the heroine who went into the garden to cut a cabbage-leaf to make an apple-pie; while yet there is no conceivable human logic so close and inexorable as her connections. How rigid, how flexible are, for instance, the laws of perspective! If one could learn to make his statements as firm and unswerving as the horizon-line, — his continuity of thought as marked, yet as unbroken, as yonder soft gradations by which the eye is lured upward from lake to wood, from wood to hill, from hill to heavens, — what more bracing tonic could literary culture demand? As it is, Art misses the parts, yet does not grasp the whole.

Literature also learns from Nature the use of materials: either to select only the choicest and rarest, or to transmute coarse to fine by skill in using. How perfect is the delicacy with which the woods and fields are kept, throughout the year! All these millions of living creatures born every season, and born to die; yet where are the dead bodies? We never see them. Buried beneath the earth by tiny nightly sextons, sunk beneath the waters, dissolved into the air, or distilled again and again as food for other organizations, — all have had their swift resurrection. Their existence blooms again in these violet-petals, glitters in the burnished beauty of these golden beetles, or enriches the veery's song. It is only out of doors that even death and decay become beautiful. The model farm, the most luxurious house, have their regions of unsightliness; but the fine chemistry of Nature is constantly clearing away all its impurities before our eyes, and yet so delicately that we never suspect the process. The most exquisite work of literary art exhibits a certain crudeness and coarseness, when we turn to it from Nature, — as the smallest cambric needle appears rough and jagged, when compared through the magnifier with the tapering fineness of the insect's sting.

Once separated from Nature, literature recedes into metaphysics, or dwindles into novels. How ignoble seems the current material of London literary life, for instance, compared with the noble simplicity which, a half-century ago, made the Lake Country an enchanted land forever! Is it worth a voyage to England to sup with Thackeray in the Pot Tavern? Compare the "enormity of pleasure" which De Quincey says Wordsworth derived from the simplest natural object, with the serious protest of Wilkie Collins against the affectation of caring about

Nature at all. "Is it not strange," says this most unhappy man, "to see how little real hold the objects of the natural world amidst which we live can gain on our hearts and minds? We go to Nature for comfort in joy and sympathy in trouble, only in books. . . . . . What share have the attractions of Nature ever had in the pleasurable or painful interests and emotions of ourselves or our friends? . . . . . There is surely a reason for this want of inborn sympathy between the creature and the creation around it."

Leslie says of "the most original landscape-painter he knew," meaning Constable, that, whenever he sat down in the fields to sketch, he endeavored to forget that he had ever seen a picture. In literature this is easy, the descriptions are so few and so faint. When Wordsworth was fourteen, he stopped one day by the wayside to observe the dark outline of an oak against the western sky; and he says that he was at that moment struck with "the infinite variety of natural appearances which had been unnoticed by the poets of any age or country," so far as he was acquainted with them, and "made a resolution to supply in some degree the deficiency." He spent a long life in studying and telling these beautiful wonders; and yet, so vast is the sum of them, they seem almost as undescribed as before, and men to be still as content with vague or conventional representations. On this continent, especially, people fancied that all must be tame and second-hand, everything long since duly analyzed and distributed and put up in appropriate quotations, and nothing left for us poor American children but a preoccupied universe. And yet Thoreau camps down by Walden Pond, and shows us that absolutely nothing in Nature has ever yet been described, — not a bird nor a berry of the woods, nor a drop of water, nor a spicula of ice, nor summer, nor winter, nor sun, nor star.

Indeed, no person can portray Nature from any slight or transient acquaintance. A reporter cannot step out between the sessions of a caucus and give a racy abstract of the landscape. It may consume the best hours of many days to certify for one's self the simplest out-door fact, but every such piece of knowledge is intellectually worth the time. Even the driest and barest book of Natural History is good and nutritious, so far as it goes, if it represents genuine acquaintance; one can find summer in January by poring over the Latin catalogues of Massachusetts plants and animals in Hitchcock's Report. The most commonplace out-door society has the same attraction. Every one of those old outlaws who haunt our New-England ponds and marshes, water-soaked and soakers of something else, — intimate with the pure fluid in that familiarity which breeds contempt, — has yet a wholesome side when you explore his knowledge of frost and freshet, pickerel and musk-rat, and is exceedingly good company while you can keep him beyond scent of the tavern. Any intelligent farmer's boy can give you some narrative of out-door observation which, so far as it goes, fulfils Milton's definition of poetry, "simple, sensuous, passionate." He may not write sonnets to the lake, but he will walk miles to bathe in it; he may not notice the sunsets, but he knows where to search for the blackbird's nest. How surprised the school-children looked, to be sure, when the Doctor of Divinity from the city tried to sentimentalize, in addressing them, about "the bobolink in the woods"! They knew that the darling of the meadow had no more personal acquaintance with the woods than was exhibited by the preacher.

But the preachers are not much worse than the authors. The prosaic Buckle, indeed, admits that the poets have in all time been consummate observers, and that their observations have been as valuable as those of the men of science; and yet we look even to the poets for very casual and occasional glimpses of Nature only, not for any continuous reflection of her glory. Thus, Chaucer is perfumed with early spring; Homer resounds like the sea; in the Greek Anthology the sun always shines on the fisherman's cottage by the beach; we associate the Vishnu Purana with lakes and lotuses, Keats with nightingales in forest dim, while the long grass waving on the lonely heath is the last memorial of the fading fame of Ossian. Of course Shakespeare's omniscience included all natural phenomena; but the rest, great or small, associate themselves with some special aspects, and not with the daily atmosphere. Coming to our own times, one must quarrel with Ruskin as taking rather the artist's view of Nature, selecting the available bits and dealing rather patronizingly with the whole; and one is tempted to charge even Emerson, as he somewhere charges Wordsworth, with not being of a temperament quite liquid and musical enough to admit the full vibration of the great harmonies. The three human foster-children who have been taken nearest into Nature's bosom, perhaps, — an odd triad, surely, for the whimsical nursing mother to select, — are Wordsworth, Bettine Brentano, and Thoreau. Is it yielding to an individual preference too far to say, that there seems almost a generic difference between these three and any others, — however wide be the specific differences among themselves, — to say, that, after all, they in their several paths have attained to an habitual intimacy with Nature, and the rest have not?

Yet what wonderful achievements have some of the fragmentary artists performed! Some of Tennyson's word-pictures, for instance, bear almost as much study as the landscape. One afternoon, last spring, I had been walking though a copse of young white birches, — their leaves scarce yet apparent, — over a ground delicate with wood-anemones, moist and mottled with dog's-tooth-violet leaves, and spangled with the delicate clusters of that shy creature, the Claytonia or Spring Beauty. All this was floored with last year's faded foliage, giving a singular bareness and whiteness to the foreground. Suddenly, as if entering a cavern, I stepped through the edge of all this, into a dark little amphitheatre beneath a hemlock-grove, where the afternoon sunlight struck broadly through the trees upon a tiny stream and a miniature swamp, — this last being intensely and luridly green, yet overlaid with the pale gray of last year's reeds, and absolutely flaming with the gayest yellow light from great clumps of cowslips. The illumination seemed perfectly weird and dazzling; the spirit of the place appeared live, wild, fantastic, almost human. Now open your Tennyson: —

"*And the wild marsh-marigold shines like fire in swamps and hollows gray.*"

Our cowslip is the English marsh-marigold.

History is a grander poetry, and it is often urged that the features of Nature in America must seem tame because they have no legendary wreaths to decorate them. It is perhaps hard for those of us who are untravelled to appreciate how densely even the ruralities of Europe are overgrown with this ivy of associations. Thus, it is fascinating to hear that the great French forests of Fontainebleau and St. Germain are full of historic trees, — the oak of Charlemagne, the oak of Clovis, of Queen Blanche, of Henri Quatre, of Sully, — the alley of Richelieu, — the rendezvous of St. Hérem, — the star of Lamballe and of the Princesses, a star being a point where several paths or roads converge. It is said that every topographical work upon these forests has turned out a history of the French monarchy. Yet surely we lose nearly as much as we gain by this subordination of imperishable beauty to the perishable memories of man. It may not be wholly unfortunate, that, in the absence of those influences which come to older nations from ruins and traditions, we must go more directly to Nature. Art may either rest upon other Art, or it may rest directly upon the original foundation; the one is easier, the other more valuable. Direct dependence on Nature leads to deeper thought, and affords the promise of far fresher results. Why should I wish to fix my study in Heidelberg Castle, when I possess the unexhausted treasures of this out-door study here?

The walls of my study are of ever-changing verdure, and its roof and floor of ever-varying blue. I never enter it without a new heaven above and new thoughts below. The lake has no lofty shores and no level ones, but a series of undulating hills, fringed with woods from end to end. The profaning axe may sometimes come near the margin, and one may hear the whetting of the scythe; but no cultivated land abuts upon the main lake, though beyond the narrow woods there are here and there glimpses of rye-fields that wave like rolling mist. Graceful islands rise from the quiet waters, — Grape Island, Grass Island, Sharp Pine Island, and the rest, baptized with simple names by departed generations of farmers, — all wooded and bushy and trailing with festoonery of vines. Here and there the banks are indented, and one may pass beneath drooping chestnut-leaves and among alder-branches into some secret sanctuary of stillness. The emerald edges of these silent tarns are starred with dandelions which have strayed here, one scarce knows how, from their foreign home; the buck-bean perchance grows in the water, or the Rhodora fixes here one of its shy camping-places, or there are whole skies of lupine on the sloping banks; — the cat-bird builds its nest beside us, the yellow-bird above, the wood-thrush sings late and the whippoorwill later, and sometimes the scarlet tanager and his golden-haired bride send a gleam of the tropics through these leafy aisles.

Sometimes I rest in a yet more secluded place amid the waters, where a little wooded island holds a small lagoon in the centre, just wide enough for the wherry to turn round. The entrance lies between two hornbeam trees, which stand close to the brink, spreading over it their thorn-like branches and their shining leaves. Within there is perfect shelter; the island forms a high circular bank, like a coral reef, and shuts out the wind and the passing boats; the surface is paved with leaves of lily and pond-weed, and the boughs above are full of song. No matter what white caps may crest the blue waters of the pond, which here widens out to its broadest reach, there is always quiet here. A few oar-strokes distant lies a dam or water-break, where the whole lake is held under control by certain distant mills, towards which a sluggish stream goes winding on through miles of water-lilies. The old gray timbers of the dam are the natural resort of every boy or boatman within their reach; some come in pursuit of pickerel, some of turtles, some of bullfrogs, some of lilies, some of bathing. It is a good place for the last desideratum, and it is well to leave here the boat tethered to the vines which overhang the cove, and perform a sacred and Oriental ablution beneath the sunny afternoon.

O radiant and divine afternoon! The poets profusely celebrate silver evenings and golden mornings; but what floods on floods of beauty steep the earth and gladden it in the first hours of day's decline! The exuberant rays reflect and multiply themselves from every leaf and blade; the cows lie upon the hillside, with their broad peaceful backs painted into the landscape; the hum of insects, "tiniest bells on the garment of silence," fills the air; the gorgeous butterflies doze upon the thistle-blooms till they almost fall from the petals; the air is full of warm fragrance from the wild-grape clusters; the grass is burning hot beneath the naked feet in sunshine, and cool as water in the shade. Diving from this overhanging beam, — for Ovid evidently meant that Midas to be cured must dive, —

"Subde caput, corpusque simul, simul elue crinem," —

one finds as kindly a reception from the water as in childish days, and as safe a shelter in the green dressing-room afterwards; and the patient wherry floats near by, in readiness for a re-embarkation.

Here a word seems needed, unprofessionally and non-technically, upon boats, — these being the sole seats provided for occupant or visitor in my out-door study. When wherries first appeared in this peaceful inland community, the novel proportions occasioned remark. Facetious by-standers inquired sarcastically whether that thing were expected to carry more than one, — plainly implying by labored emphasis that it would occasionally be seen tenanted by even less than that number. Transcendental friends inquired, with more refined severity, if the proprietor expected to *meditate* in that thing? This doubt at least seemed legitimate. Meditation seems to belong to sailing rather than rowing; there is something so gentle and unintrusive in gliding effortless beneath overhanging branches and along the trailing edges of clematis thickets; — what a privilege of fairy-land is this noiseless prow, looking in and out of one flowery cove after another, scarcely stirring the turtle from his log, and leaving no wake behind! It seemed as if all the process of rowing had too much noise and bluster, and as if the sharp slender wherry, in particular, were rather too pert and dapper to win the confidence of the woods and waters. Time has dispelled the fear. As I rest poised upon the oars above some submerged shallow, diamonded with ripple-broken sunbeams, the fantastic Notonecta or water-boatman rests upon his oars below, and I see that his proportions anticipated the wherry, as honeycombs antedated the problem of the hexagonal cell. While one of us rests, so does the other; and when one shoots away rapidly above the water, the other does the same beneath. For the time, as our motions seem the same, so with our motives, — my enjoyment certainly not less, with the conveniences of humanity thrown in.

But the sun is declining low. The club-boats are out, and from island to island in the distance these shafts of youthful life shoot swiftly across. There races some swift Atalanta, with no apple to fall in her path but some soft and spotted oak-apple from an overhanging tree; there the Phantom, with a crew white and ghostlike in the distance, glimmers in and out behind the headlands, while yonder wherry glides lonely across the smooth expanse. The voices of all these oarsmen are dim and almost inaudible, being so far away; but one would scarcely wish that distance should annihilate the ringing laughter of these joyous girls, who come gliding, in a safe and heavy boat, they and some blue dragon-flies together, around yonder wooded point.

Many a summer afternoon have I rowed joyously with these same maidens beneath these steep and garlanded shores; many a time have they pulled the heavy four-oar, with me as coxswain at the helm, — the said patient steersman being ofttimes insulted by classical allusions from rival boats, satirically comparing him to an indolent Venus drawn by doves, while the oarswomen, in turn, were likened to Minerva with her feet upon a tortoise. Many were the disasters in the earlier days of feminine training; — first of toilet, — straw hats blowing away, hair coming down, hair-pins strewing the floor of the boat, gloves commonly happening to be off at the precise moment of starting, and trials of speed impaired by somebody's oar catching in somebody's dress-pocket. Then the actual difficulties of handling the long and heavy oars, — the first essays at feathering, with a complicated splash of air and water, as when a wild duck, in rising, swims and flies together, and uses neither element handsomely, — the occasional pulling of a particularly vigorous stroke through the atmosphere alone, and at other times the compensating disappearance of nearly the whole oar beneath the liquid surface, as if some Uncle Kühleborn had grasped it, while our Undine by main strength tugged it from the beguiling wave. But with what triumphant abundance of merriment were these preliminary disasters repaid, and how soon outgrown! What "time" we sometimes made, when nobody happened to be near with a watch, and how successfully we tossed oars in saluting, when the world looked on from a picnic! We had our applauses, too. To be sure, owing to the age and dimensions of the original barge, we could not command such a burst of enthusiasm as when the young men shot by us in their race-boat; but then, as one of the girls justly remarked, we remained longer in sight.

And many a day, since promotion to a swifter craft, have they rowed with patient stroke down the lovely lake, still attended by their guide, philosopher, and coxswain, — along banks where herds of young birch-trees overspread the sloping valley, and ran down in a blaze of sunshine to the rippling water, — or through the Narrows, where some breeze rocked the boat till trailing shawls and ribbons were water-soaked, and the bold little foam would even send a daring drop over the gunwale, to play at ocean, — or to Davis's Cottage, where a whole parterre of lupines bloomed to the water's edge, as if relics of some ancient garden-bower of a forgotten race, — or to the dam by Lily Pond, there to hunt among the stones for snakes' eggs, each empty shell cut crosswise, where the young creatures had made their first fierce bite into the universe outside, — or to some island, where white violets bloomed fragrant and lonely, separated by relentless breadths of water from their shore-born sisters, until mingled in their visitors' bouquets, — then up the lake homeward again at nightfall, the boat all decked with clematis, clethra, laurel, azalea, or water-lilies, while purple sunset clouds turned forth their golden linings for drapery above our heads, and then, unrolling, sent northward long roseate wreaths to outstrip our loitering speed, and reach the floating bridge before us.

It is nightfall now. One by one the birds grow silent, and the soft dragon-flies, children of the day, are fluttering noiselessly to their rest beneath the under sides of drooping leaves. From shadowy coves the evening air is thrusting forth a thin film of mist to spread a white floor above the waters. The gathering darkness deepens the quiet of the lake, and bids us, at least for this time, to forsake it. "*De soir fontaines, de matin montaignes,*" says the old French proverb, — Morning for labor, evening for repose.

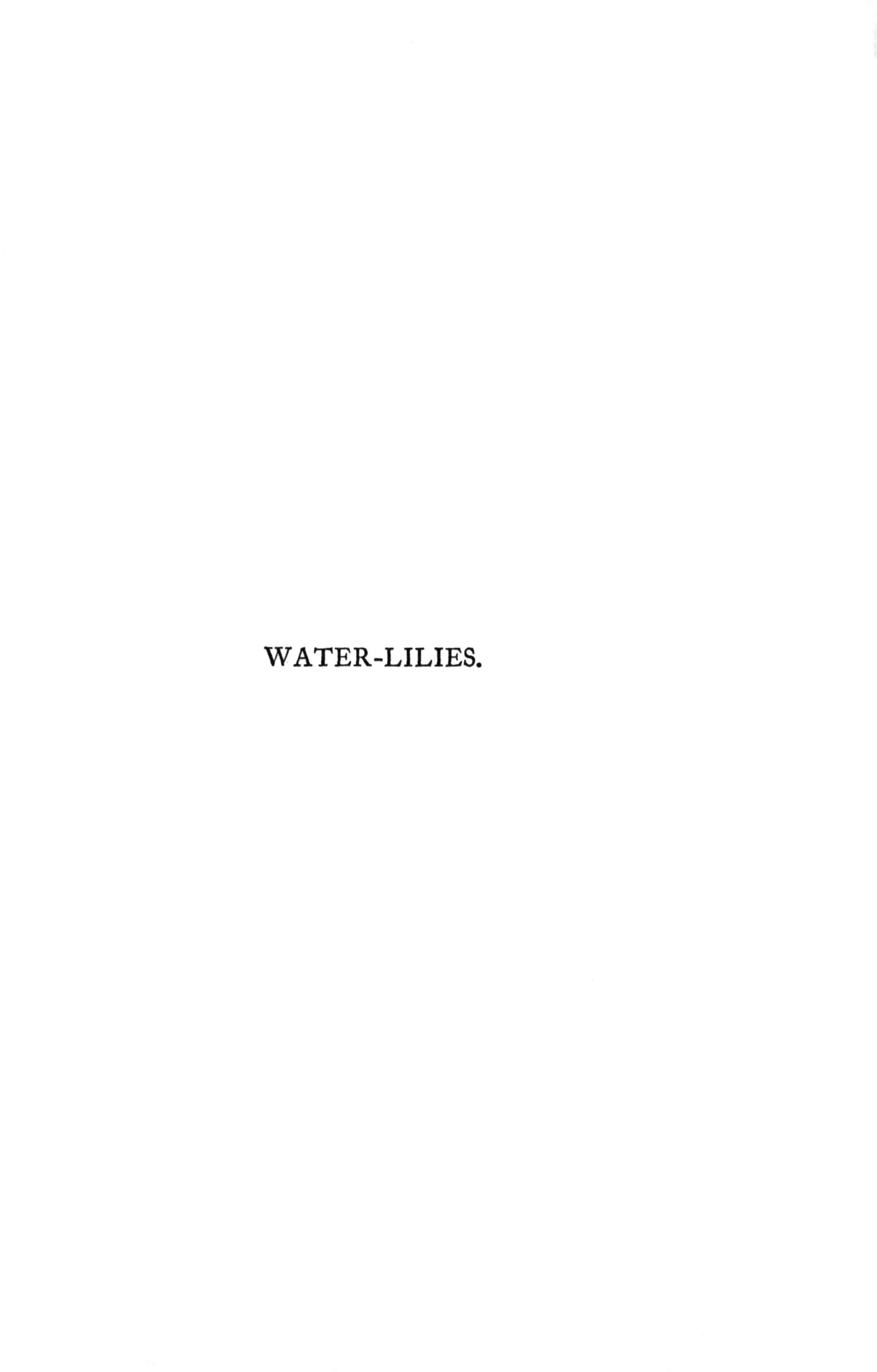

WATER-LILIES.

WATER-LILIES.

THE inconstant April mornings drop showers or sunbeams over the glistening lake, while far beneath its surface a murky mass disengages itself from the muddy bottom, and rises slowly through the waves. The tasselled alder-branches droop above it; the last year's blackbird's nest swings over it in the grape-vine; the newly-opened Hepaticas and Epigæas on the neighboring bank peer down modestly to look for it; the water-skater (Gerris) pauses on the surface near it, casting on the shallow bottom the odd shadow of his feet, like three pairs of boxing-gloves; the Notonecta, or water-boatman, rows round and round it, sometimes on his breast, sometimes on his back; queer caddis-worms trail their self-made homesteads of leaves or twigs beside it; the Dytiscus, dorbug of the water, blunders clumsily against it; the tadpole wriggles his stupid way to it, and rests upon it, meditating of future frogdom; the passing wild-duck dives and nibbles at it; the mink and muskrat brush it with their soft fur; the spotted turtle slides over it; the slow larvæ of gauzy dragon-flies cling sleepily to its sides and await their change: all these fair or uncouth creatures feel, through the dim waves, the blessed longing of spring; and yet not one of them dreams that within that murky mass there lies a treasure too white and beautiful to be yet intrusted to the waves, and that for many a day the bud must yearn toward the surface, before, aspiring above it, as mortals to heaven, it meets the sunshine with the answering beauty of the Water-Lily.

Days and weeks have passed away; the wild-duck has flown onward, to dive for his luncheon in some remoter lake; the tadpoles have made themselves legs, with which they have vanished; the caddis-worms have sealed themselves up in their cylinders, and emerged again as winged insects; the dragon-flies have crawled up the water-reeds, and, clinging with heads upturned, have undergone the change which symbolizes immortality; the world is transformed from spring to summer; the lily-buds are opened into glossy leaf and radiant flower, and we have come for the harvest.

We visitors lodged, last night, in the old English phrase, "at the sign of the Oak and Star." Wishing, not, indeed, like the ancient magicians, to gather magic berry and bud before sunrise, but at least to see these treasures of the lake in their morning hour, we camped last night on a little island, which one tall tree almost covers with its branches, while a dense undergrowth of young chestnuts and birches fills all the intervening space, touching the water all around the circular, shelving shore. Yesterday was hot, but the night was cool, and we kindled a gypsy fire of twigs, less for warmth than for society. The first gleam made the dark, lonely islet into a cheering home, turned the protecting tree to a starlit roof, and the chestnut-sprays to illuminated walls. To us, lying beneath their shelter, every fresh flickering of the fire kindled the leaves into brightness and banished into dark interstices the lake and sky; then the fire died into embers, the leaves faded into solid darkness in their turn, and water and heavens showed light and close and near, until fresh twigs caught fire and the blaze came up again. Rising to look forth, at intervals, during the peaceful hours, — for it is the worst feature of a night out-doors, that sleeping seems such a waste of time, — we watched the hilly and wooded shores of the lake sink into gloom and glimmer into dawn again, amid the low plash of waters and the noises of the night.

Precisely at half past three, a song-sparrow above our heads gave one liquid trill, so inexpressibly sudden and delicious, that it seemed to set to music every atom of freshness and fragrance that Nature held; then the spell was broken, and the whole shore and lake were vocal with song. Joining in this jubilee of morning, we were early in motion; bathing and breakfast, though they seemed indisputably in accordance with the instincts of the Universe, yet did not detain us long, and we were promptly on our way to Lily Pond. Will the reader join us?

It is one of those summer days when a veil of mist gradually burns away before the intense sunshine, and the sultry morning only plays at coolness, and that with its earliest visitors alone. But we are before the sunlight, though not before the sunrise, and can watch the pretty game of alternating mist and shine. Stray gleams of glory lend their trailing magnificence to the tops of chestnut-trees, floating vapors raise the outlines of the hills and make mystery of the wooded islands, and, as we glide through the placid water, we can sing, with the Chorus in the "Ion" of Euripides, "O immense and brilliant air, resound with our cries of joy!"

Almost every town has its Lily Pond, dear to boys

and maidens, and partially equalizing, by its annual delights, the presence or absence of other geographical advantages. Ours is accessible from the larger lake only by taking the skiff over a narrow embankment, which protects our fairy-land by its presence, and eight distant factories by its dam. Once beyond it, we are in a realm of dark Lethean water, utterly unlike the sunny depths of the main lake. Hither the water-lilies have retreated, to a domain of their own. In the bosom of these shallow waves, there stand hundreds of submerged and dismasted roots, still upright, spreading their vast, uncouth limbs like enormous spiders beneath the surface. They are remnants of border wars with the axe, vegetable Witheringtons, still fighting on their stumps, but gradually sinking into the soft ooze, and ready, perhaps, when a score of centuries has piled two more strata of similar remains in mud above them, to furnish foundations for a newer New Orleans; that city having been lately discovered to be thus supported.

The present decline in the manufacturing business is clear revenue to the water-lilies, and these ponds are higher than usual, because the idle mills do not draw them off. But we may notice, in observing the shores, that peculiar charm of water, that, whether its quantity be greater or less, its grace is the same; it makes its own boundary in lake or river, and where its edge is, there seems the natural and permanent margin. And the same natural fitness, without reference to mere quantity, extends to its flowery children. Before us lie islands and continents of lilies, acres of charms, whole, vast, unbroken surfaces of stainless whiteness. And yet, as we approach them, every islanded cup that floats in lonely dignity, apart from the multitude, appears as perfect in itself, couched in white expanded perfection, its reflection taking a faint glory of pink that is scarcely perceptible in the flower. As we glide gently among them, the air grows fragrant, and a stray breeze flaps the leaves, as if to welcome us. Each floating flower becomes suddenly a ship at anchor, or rather seems beating up against the summer wind, in a regatta of blossoms.

Early as it is in the day, the greater part of the flowers are already expanded. Indeed, that experience of Thoreau's, of watching them open in the first sunbeams, rank by rank, is not easily obtained, unless perhaps in a narrow stream, where the beautiful slumberers are more regularly marshalled. In our lake, at least, they open irregularly, though rapidly. But, this morning, many linger as buds, while others peer up, in half-expanded beauty, beneath the lifted leaves, frolicsome as Pucks or baby-nymphs. As you raise the leaf, in such cases, it is impossible not to imagine that a pair of tiny hands have upheld it, and that the pretty head will dip down again, and disappear. Others, again, have expanded all but the inmost pair of white petals, and these spring apart at the first touch of the finger on the stem. Some spread vast vases of fragrance, six or seven inches in diameter, while others are small and delicate, with petals like fine lace-work. Smaller still, we sometimes pass a flotilla of infant leaves, an inch in diameter. All these grow from the dark water, — and the blacker it is, the fairer their whiteness shows. But your eye follows the stem often vainly into those sombre depths, and vainly seeks to behold Sabrina fair, sitting with her twisted braids of lilies, beneath the glassy, cool, but not translucent wave. Do not start, when, in such an effort, only your own dreamy face looks back upon you, beyond the gunwale of the reflected boat, and you find that you float double, self and shadow.

Let us rest our paddles, and look round us, while the idle motion sways our light skiff onward, now half embayed among the lily-pads, now lazily gliding over intervening gulfs. There is a great deal going on in these waters and their fringing woods and meadows. All the summer long, the pond is bordered with successive walls of flowers. In early spring emerge the yellow catkins of the swamp-willow, first; then the long tassels of the graceful alders expand and droop, till they weep their yellow dust upon the water; then come the birch-blossoms, more tardily; then the downy leaves and white clusters of the medlar or shad-bush (*Amelanchier Canadensis* of Gray); these dropping, the roseate chalices of the mountain-laurel open; as they fade into melancholy brown, the sweet Azalea uncloses; and before its last honeyed blossom has trailed down, dying, from the stem, the more fragrant Clethra starts out above, the button-bush thrusts forth its merry face amid wild roses, and the Clematis waves its sprays of beauty. Mingled with these grow, lower, the spiræas, white and pink, yellow touch-me-not, fresh white arrowhead, bright blue vervain and skullcap, dull snakehead, gay monkey-flower, coarse eupatoriums, milkweeds, golden-rods, asters, thistles, and a host beside. Beneath, the brilliant scarlet cardinal-flower begins to palisade the moist shores; and after its superb reflection has passed away from the waters, the grotesque witch-hazel flares out its narrow yellow petals amidst the October leaves, and so ends the floral year. There is not a week during all these months, when one cannot stand in the boat and wreathe garlands of blossoms from the shores.

These all crowd around the brink, and watch, day and

night, the opening and closing of the water-lilies. Meanwhile, upon the waters, our queen keeps her chosen court, nor can one of these mere land-loving blossoms touch the hem of her garment. In truth, she bears no sister near her throne. There is but this one species among us, *Nymphæa odorata.* The beautiful little rose-colored *Nymphæa sanguinea,* which once adorned the Botanic Garden at Cambridge, was merely an occasional variety of costume. She has, indeed, an English half-sister, *Nymphæa alba,* less beautiful, less fragrant, but keeping more fashionable hours, — not opening (according to Linnæus) till seven, nor closing till four. And she has a humble cousin, the yellow Nuphar, who keeps commonly aloof, as becomes a poor relation, though created from the self-same mud, — a fact which Hawthorne has beautifully moralized. The prouder Nelumbium, a second-cousin, lineal descendant of the sacred bean of Pythagoras, has fallen to an obscurer position, and dwells, like a sturdy democrat, in the Far West.

But, undisturbed, the water-lily reigns on, with her retinue around her. The tall pickerel-weed (Pontederia) is her gentleman-usher, gorgeous in blue and gold through July, somewhat rusty in August. The water-shield (Hydropeltis) is chief maid-of-honor; a high-born lady she, not without royal blood indeed, but with rather a bend sinister; not precisely beautiful, but very fastidious; encased over her whole person with a gelatinous covering, literally a starched duenna. Sometimes she is suspected of conspiring to drive her mistress from the throne; for we have observed certain slow watercourses where the leaves of the water-lily have been almost wholly replaced, in a series of years, by the similar, but smaller, leaves of the water-shield. More rarely seen is the slender Utricularia, a dainty maiden, whose light feet scarce touch the water, — with the still more delicate floating white Water-Ranunculus, and the shy Villarsia, whose submerged flowers merely peep one day above the surface and then close again forever. Then there are many humbler attendants, Potamogetons or pond-weeds. And here float little emissaries from the dominions of land; for the fallen florets of the Viburnum drift among the lily-pads, with mast-like stamens erect, sprinkling the water with a strange beauty, and cheating us with the promise of a new aquatic flower.

These are the still life of this sequestered nook; but it is in fact a crowded thoroughfare. No tropic jungle more swarms with busy existence than these midsummer waters and their bushy banks. The warm and humming air is filled with insect sounds, ranging from the murmur of invisible gnats and midges, to the impetuous whirring of the great Libellulæ, large almost as swallows, and hawking high in air for their food. Swift butterflies glance by, moths flutter, flies buzz, grasshoppers and katydids pipe their shrill notes, sharp as the edges of the sunbeams. Busy bees go humming past, straight as arrows, express-freight-trains from one blossoming copse to another. Showy wasps of many species fume uselessly about, in gallant uniforms, wasting an immense deal of unnecessary anger on the sultry universe. Graceful, stingless Sphexes and Ichneumon-flies emulate their bustle, without their weapons. Delicate lady-birds come and go to the milkweeds, spotted almost as regularly as if Nature had decided to number the species, like policemen or hack-drivers, from one to twenty. Elegant little Lepturæ fly with them, so gay and airy, they hardly seem like beetles. Phryganeæ (*nés* caddis-worms), lace-flies, and long-tailed Ephemeræ flutter more heavily by. On the large alder-flowers clings the superb *Desmocerus palliatus*, beautiful as a tropical insect, with his steel-blue armor and his golden cloak (*pallium*) above his shoulders, grandest knight on this Field of the Cloth of Gold. The countless fire-flies which spangled the evening mist now only crawl sleepily, daylight creatures, with the lustre buried in their milky bodies. More wholly children of night, the soft, luxurious Sphinxes (or hawk-moths) come not here; fine ladies of the insect world, their home is among gardens and green-houses, late and languid by day, but all night long upon the wing, dancing in the air with unwearied muscles till long past midnight, and supping on honey at last. They come not; but the nobler butterflies soar above us, stoop a moment to the water, and then with a few lazy wavings of their sumptuous wings float far over the oak-trees to the woods they love.

All these hover near the water-lily; but its special parasites are an enamelled beetle (*Donacia metallica*) which keeps house permanently in the flower, and a few smaller ones which tenant the surface of the leaves,— larva, pupa, and perfect insect, forty feeding like one, and each leading its whole earthly career on this floating island of perishable verdure. The "beautiful blue damsel-flies" alight also in multitudes among them, so fearless that they perch with equal readiness on our boat or paddle, and so various that two adjacent ponds will sometimes be haunted by two distinct sets of species. In the water, among the leaves, little shining whirlwigs wheel round and round, fifty joining in the dance, till, at the slightest alarm, they whirl away to some safer ball-room, and renew the merriment. On every floating log, as we approach it, there is a convention of turtles, sitting in calm debate, like mailed barons, till, as we draw near, they plump into the water, and paddle away for some subaqueous Runnymede. Beneath, the shy and stately pickerel vanishes at a glance, shoals of minnows glide, black and bearded pouts frisk aimlessly, soft water-newts hang poised without motion, and slender pickerel-frogs cease occasionally their submerged croaking, and, darting to the surface with swift vertical strokes, gulp a mouthful of fresh air, and down again to renew the moist soliloquy.

Time would fail us to tell of the feathered life around us, — the blackbirds that build securely in these thickets, the stray swallows that dip their wings in the quiet waters, and the kingfishers that still bring, as the ancients fabled, halcyon days. Yonder stands, against the shore, a bittern, motionless in that wreath of mist which makes his long-legged person almost as dim as his far-off booming by night. There poises a hawk, before sweeping down to some chosen bough in the dense forest; and there fly a pair of blue-jays, screaming, from tree to tree. As for wild quadrupeds, the race is almost passed away. Far to the north, indeed, the great moose still browses on the lily-pads, and the shy beaver nibbles them; but here the few lingering four-footed creatures only haunt, but do not graze upon, these floating pastures. Eyes more favored than ours may yet chance to spy an otter in this still place; there by the shore are the small footprints of a mink; that dark thing disappearing in the waters yonder, a soft mass of drowned fur, is a "musquash." Later in the season, a mound of earth will be his winter dwelling-place; and those myriad muscle-shells at the water's edge are the remnant of his banquets, — once banquets for the Indians, too.

But we must return to our lilies. There is no sense of wealth like floating in this archipelago of white and green. The emotions of avarice become almost demoralizing. Every flower bears a fragrant California in its bosom, and you feel impoverished at the thought of leaving one behind. But after the first half-hour of eager grasping, one becomes fastidious, rather avoids those on which the wasps and flies have alighted, and seeks only the stainless. But handle them tenderly, as if you loved them. Do not grasp at the open flower as if it were a peony or a hollyhock, for then it will come off, stalkless, in your hand, and you will cast it blighted upon the water; but coil your thumb and second finger affectionately around it, press the extended forefinger firmly to the stem below, and, with one steady pull, you will secure a long and delicate stalk, fit to twine around the graceful head of your beloved, as the Hindoo goddess of beauty encircled with a Lotus the brow of Rama.

Consider the lilies. All over our rural watercourses, at midsummer, float these cups of snow. They are Nature's symbols of coolness. They suggest to us the white garments of their Oriental worshippers. They come with the white roses, and prepare the way for the white lilies of the garden. The white doe of Rylstone and Andrew Marvell's fawn might fitly bathe amid their beauties. Yonder steep bank slopes down to the lake-side, one solid mass of pale pink laurel, but, once upon the water, a purer tint prevails. The pink fades into a lingering flush, and the white creature floats peerless, set in green without and gold within. That bright circle of stamens is the very ring with which Doges once wedded the Adriatic; Venice has lost it, but it dropped into the water-lily's bosom, and there it rests forever. So perfect in form, so redundant in beauty, so delicate, so spotless, so fragrant, — what presumptuous lover ever dared, in his most enamored hour, to liken his mistress to a water-lily? No human Blanche or Lilian was ever so fair as that.

The water-lily comes of an ancient and sacred family of white-robed priests. They assisted at the most momentous religious ceremonies, from the beginning of recorded time. The Egyptian Lotus was a sacred plant; it was dedicated to Harpocrates and to the god Nofr Atmoo, — *Nofr* meaning *good,* whence the name of our yellow lily, Nuphar. But the true Egyptian flower was *Nymphæa Lotus,* though *Nymphæa cærulea,* Moore's "blue water-lilies," can be traced on the sculptures also. It was cultivated in tanks in the gardens; it was the chief material for festal wreaths; a single bud hung over the forehead of many a queenly dame; and the sculptures represent the weary flowers as dropping from the heated hands of belles, in the later hours of the feast. Rock softly on the waters, fair lilies! your Eastern kindred have rocked on the stormier bosom of Cleopatra. The Egyptian Lotus was, moreover, the emblem of the sacred Nile, — as the Hindoo species, of the sacred Ganges; and each was held the symbol of the creation of the world from the waters. The sacred bull Apis was wreathed with its garlands; there were niches for water, to place it among tombs; it was carved in the capitals of columns; it was represented on plates and vases; the sculptures show it in many sacred uses, even as a burnt-offering; Isis holds it; and the god Nilus still binds a wreath of water-lilies around the throne of Memnon.

From Egypt the Lotus was carried to Assyria, and Layard found it among fir-cones and honeysuckles on the later sculptures of Nineveh. The Greeks dedicated it to the nymphs, whence the name *Nymphæa.* Nor did the Romans disregard it, though the Lotus to which Ovid's nymph Lotis was changed, *servato nomine,* was a tree, and not a flower. Still different a thing was the en chanted stem of the Lotus-eaters of Herodotus, which prosaic botanists have reduced to the *Zizyphus Lotus* found by Mungo Park, translating also the yellow Lotus-dust into a mere "farina, tasting like sweet gingerbread."

But in the Lotus of Hindostan we find our flower again, and the Oriental sacred books are cool with water-lilies. Open the Vishnu Purana at any page, and it is a *Sortes Lilianæ.* The orb of the earth is Lotus-shaped, and is upborne by the tusks of Vesava, as if he had been sporting in a lake where the leaves and blossoms float. Brahma, first incarnation of Vishnu, creator of the world, was born from a Lotus; so was Sri or Lakshmu, the Hindoo Venus, goddess of beauty and prosperity, protectress of womanhood, whose worship guards the house from all danger. "Seated on a full-blown Lotus, and holding a Lotus in her hand, the goddess Sri, radiant with beauty, rose from the waves." The Lotus is the chief ornament of the subterranean Eden, Patala, and the holy mountain Meru is thought to be shaped like its seed-vessel, larger at summit than at base. When the heavenly Urvasi fled from her earthly spouse, Purúvavas, he found her sporting with four nymphs of heaven, in a lake beautified with the Lotus. When the virtuous Prahlada was burned at the stake, he cried to his cruel father, "The fire burneth me not, and all around I behold the face of the sky, cool and fragrant with beds of Lotus-flowers!" Above all, the graceful history of the transformations of Krishna is everywhere hung with these fresh chaplets. Every successive maiden whom the deity wooes is Lotus-eyed,

Lotus-mouthed, or Lotus-cheeked, and the youthful hero wears always a Lotus-wreath. Also "the clear sky was bright with the autumnal moon, and the air fragrant with the perfume of the wild water-lily, in whose buds the clustering bees were murmuring their song."

Elsewhere we find fuller details. "In the primordial state of the world, the rudimental universe, submerged in water, reposed on the bosom of the Eternal. Brahma, the architect of the world, poised on a Lotus-leaf, floated upon the waters, and all that he was able to discern with his eight eyes was water and darkness. Amid scenes so ungenial and dismal, the god sank into a profound reverie, when he thus soliloquized: 'Who am I? Whence am I?' In this state of abstraction Brahma continued during the period of a century and a half of the gods, without apparent benefit or a solution of his inquiries, — a circumstance which caused him great uneasiness of mind." It is a comfort, however, to know that subsequently a voice came to him, on which he rose, "seated himself upon the Lotus in an attitude of contemplation, and reflected upon the Eternal, who soon appeared to him in the form of a man with a thousand heads," — a questionable exchange for his Lotus-solitude.

This is Brahminism; but the other great form of Oriental religion has carried the same fair symbol with it. One of the Bibles of the Buddhists is named "The White Lotus of the Good Law." A pious Nepaulese bowed in reverence before a vase of lilies which perfumed the study of Sir William Jones. At sunset in Thibet, the French missionaries tell us, every inhabitant of every village prostrates himself in the public square, and the holy invocation, "O, the gem in the Lotus!" goes murmuring over hill and valley, like the sound of many bees.

It is no unmeaning phrase, but an utterance of ardent desire to be absorbed into that Brahma whose emblem is the sacred flower. This mystic formula or "mani" is imprinted on the pavement of the streets, it floats on flags from the temples, and the wealthy Buddhists maintain sculptor-missionaries, Old Mortalities of the water-lily, who, wandering to distant lands, carve the blessed words upon cliff and stone.

Having got thus far into Orientalism, we can hardly expect to get out again without some slight entanglement in philology. Lily-pads. Whence *pads?* No other leaf is identified with that singular monosyllable. Has our floating Lotus-leaf any connection with padding, or with a footpad? with the ambling pad of an abbot, or a paddle, or a paddock, or a padlock? with many-domèd Padua proud, or with St. Patrick? Is the name derived from the Anglo-Saxon *paad* or *petthian*, or the Greek πατέω? All the etymologists are silent; Tooke and Richardson ignore the problem; and of the innumerable pamphlets in the Worcester and Webster Controversy, loading the tables of school-committee-men, not one ventures to grapple with the lily-pad.

But was there ever a philological trouble for which the Sanscrit could not afford at least a conjectural cure? A dictionary of that extremely venerable tongue is an ostrich's stomach, which can crack the hardest etymological nut. The Sanscrit name for the Lotus is simply *Padma.* The learned Brahmins call the Egyptian deities Padma Devi, or Lotus-Gods; the second of the eighteen Hindoo Puranas is styled the Padma Purana, because it treats of the "epoch when the world was a golden Lotus"; and the sacred incantation which goes murmuring through Thibet is "Om mani padme houm." It would be singular, if upon these delicate floating leaves a fragment of our earliest vernacular has been borne down to us, so that here the school-boy is more learned than the *savans.*

This lets us down easily to the more familiar uses of this plant divine. By the Nile, in early days, the water-lily was good not merely for devotion, but for diet. "From the seeds of the Lotus," said Pliny, "the Egyptians make bread." The Hindoos still eat the seeds, roasted in sand; also the stalks and roots. In South America, from the seeds of the Victoria (*Nymphæa Victoria,* now *Victoria Regia*) a farina is made, preferred to that of the finest wheat, — Bonpland even suggesting to our reluctant imagination Victoria-pies. But the European species are used, so far as is reported, only in dyeing, and as food (if the truth be told) of swine. Our own water-lily is rather more powerful in its uses; the root contains tannin and gallic acid, and a decoction of it "gives a black precipitate, with sulphate of iron." It graciously consents to become an astringent, and a styptic, and a poultice, and, banished from all other temples, still lingers in those of Æsculapius.

The botanist also finds his special satisfactions in the flower. It has some strange peculiarities of structure. So loose is the internal distribution of its tissues, that it was for some time held doubtful to which of the two great vegetable divisions, exogenous or endogenous, it belonged. Its petals, moreover, furnish the best example of the gradual transition of petals into stamens, — illustrating that wonderful law of identity which is the great discovery of modern science. Every child knows this peculiarity of the water-lily, but the extent of it seems to vary with season and locality, and sometimes one finds a succession of flowers almost entirely free from this confusion of organs.

The reader may not care to learn that the order of Nymphæaceæ "differs from Ranunculaceæ in the consolidation of its carpels, from Papaveraceæ in the placentation not being parietal, and from Nelumbiaceæ in the want of a large truncated disc containing monospermous achenia"; but they may like to know that the water-lily has relations on land, in all gradations of society, from poppy to magnolia, and yet does not conform its habits precisely to those of any of them. Its great black roots, sometimes as large as a man's arm, form a network at the bottom of the water. Its stem floats, an airy four-celled tube, adapting itself to the depth, and stiff in shallows, like the stalk of the yellow lily: and it contracts and curves downward when seed-time approaches. The leaves show beneath the magnifier beautiful adaptations of structure. They are not, like those of land-plants, constructed with deep veins to receive the rain and conduct it to the stem, but are smooth and glossy, and of even surface. The leaves of land-vegetation have also thousands of little breathing-pores, principally on the under side: the apple-leaf, for instance, has twenty-four thousand to a square inch. But here they are fewer; they are wholly on the upper side, and, whereas in other cases they open or shut according to the moisture of the atmosphere, here the greedy leaves, secure of moisture, scarcely deign to close them. Nevertheless, even these give some recognition of hygrometric necessities, and, though living on the water, and not merely christened with dewdrops like other leaves, but baptized by immersion all the time, they are yet known to suffer in drought and to take pleasure in the rain.

After speaking of the various kindred of the water-lily, it would be wrong to leave our fragrant subject without due mention of its most magnificent, most lovely relative, at first claimed even as its twin sister, and classed as a Nymphæa. I once lived near neighbor to a Victoria Regia. Nothing in the world of vegetable existence has such a human interest. The charm is not in the mere size of the plant, which disappoints everybody, as Niagara does, when tried by that sole standard. The leaves of the Victoria, indeed, attain a diameter of six feet; the largest flowers, of twenty-three inches, — four times the size of the largest of our water-lilies. But it is not the measurements of the Victoria, it is its life which fascinates. It is not a thing merely of dimensions, nor merely of beauty, but a creature of vitality and motion. Those vast leaves expand and change almost visibly. They have been known to grow half an inch an hour, eight inches a day. Rising one day from the water, a mere clenched mass of yellow prickles, a leaf is transformed the next day to a crimson salver, gorgeously tinted on its upturned rim. Then it spreads into a raft of green, armed with long thorns, and supported by a framework of ribs and cross-pieces, an inch thick, and so substantial, that the Brazil Indians, while gathering the seed-vessels, place their young children on the leaves; — *yrupe*, or water-platter, they call the accommodating plant. But even these expanding leaves are not the glory of the Victoria; the glory is in the opening of the flower.

I have sometimes looked in, for a passing moment, at the green-house, its dwelling-place, during the period of flowering, — and then stayed for more than an hour, unable to leave the fascinating scene. After the strange flower-bud has reared its dark head from the placid tank, moving it a little, uneasily, like some imprisoned water-creature, it pauses for a moment in a sort of dumb despair. Then trembling again, and collecting all its powers, it thrusts open, with an indignant jerk, the rough calyx-leaves, and the beautiful disrobing begins. The firm, white, central cone, first so closely infolded, quivers a little, and swiftly, before your eyes, the first of the hundred petals detaches its delicate edges, and springs back, opening towards the water, while its white reflection opens to meet it from below. Many moments of repose follow, — you watch, — another petal trembles, detaches, springs open, and is still. Then another, and another, and another. Each movement is so quiet, yet so decided, so living, so human, that the radiant creature seems a Musidora of the water, and you almost blush with a sense of guilt, in gazing on that peerless privacy. As petal by petal slowly opens, there still stands the central cone of snow, a glacier, an alp, a jungfrau, while each avalanche of whiteness seems the last. Meanwhile a strange rich odor fills the air, and Nature seems to concentrate all fascinations and claim all senses for this jubilee of her darling.

So pass the enchanted moments of the evening, till the fair thing pauses at last, and remains for hours unchanged. In the morning, one by one, those white petals close again, shutting all their beauty in, and you watch through the short sleep for the period of waking. Can this bright transfigured creature appear again, in the same chaste loveliness? Your fancy can scarcely trust it, fearing some disastrous change; and your fancy is too true a prophet. Come again, after the second day's opening, and you start at the transformation which one hour has secretly produced. Can this be the virgin Victoria, — this thing of crimson passion, this pile of pink and yellow, relaxed, expanded, voluptuous, lolling languidly upon the water, never to rise again? In this short time every tint of every petal is transformed; it is gorgeous in beauty, but it is "Hebe turned to Magdalen."

Such is the Victoria Regia. But our rustic water-lily, our innocent Nymphæa, never claiming such a hot-house glory, never drooping into such a blush, blooms on placidly in the quiet waters, till she modestly folds her leaves for the last time, and bows her head beneath the surface forever. Next year she lives for us only in her children, fair and pure as herself.

Nay, not alone in them, but also in memory. The fair vision will not fade from us, though the paddle has dipped its last crystal drop from the waves, and the boat is drawn upon the shore. We may yet visit many lovely and lonely places, — meadows thick with violet, or the homes of the shy Rhodora, or those sloping forest-haunts where the slight Linnæa hangs its twin-born heads, — but no scene will linger on our vision like this annual Feast of the Lilies. On scorching mountains, amid raw prairie-winds, or upon the regal ocean, the white pageant shall come back to memory again, with all the luxury of summer heats, and all the fragrant coolness that can relieve them. We shall fancy ourselves again among these fleets of anchored lilies, — again, like Urvasi, sporting amid the Lake of Lotuses.

For that which is remembered is often more vivid than that which is seen. The eye paints better in the presence, the heart in the absence, of the object most dear. "He who longs after beautiful Nature can best describe her," said Bettine; "he who is in the midst of her loveliness can only lie down and enjoy." It enhances the truth of the poet's verses, that he writes them in his study. Absence is the very air of passion, and all the best description is *in memoriam.* As with our human beloved, when the graceful presence is with us, we cannot analyze or describe, but merely possess, and only after its departure can it be portrayed by our yearning desires; so is it with Nature: only in losing her do we gain the power to describe her, and we are introduced to Art, as we are to Eternity, by the dropping away of our companions.

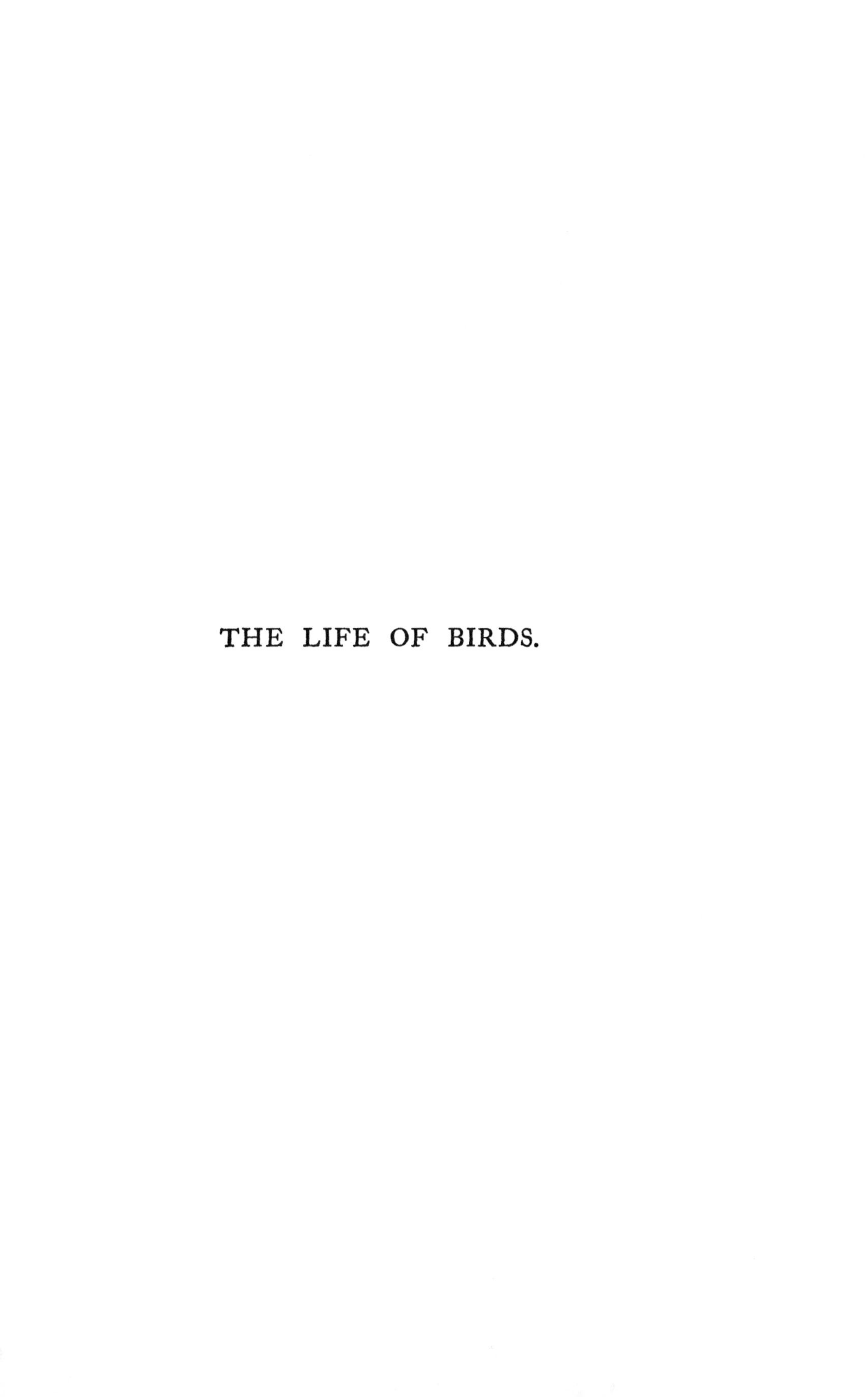

THE LIFE OF BIRDS.

THE LIFE OF BIRDS.

WHEN one thinks of a bird, one fancies a soft, swift, aimless, joyous thing, full of nervous energy and arrowy motions, — a song with wings. So remote from ours their mode of existence, they seem accidental exiles from an unknown globe, banished where none can understand their language; and men only stare at their darting, inexplicable ways, as at the gyrations of the circus. Watch their little traits for hours, and it only tantalizes curiosity. Every man's secret is penetrable, if his neighbor be sharp-sighted. Dickens, for instance, can take a poor condemned wretch, like Fagin, whose emotions neither he nor his reader has experienced, and can paint him in colors that seem made of the soul's own atoms, so that each beholder feels as if he, personally, had been the man. But this bird that hovers and alights beside me, peers up at me, takes its food, then looks again, attitudinizing, jerking, flirting its tail, with a thousand inquisitive and fantastic motions, — although I have power to grasp it in my hand and crush its life out, yet I cannot gain its secret thus, and the centre of its consciousness is really farther from mine than the remotest planetary orbit. "We do not steadily bear in mind," says Darwin, with a noble scientific humility, "how profoundly ignorant we are of the condition of existence of every animal."

What "sympathetic penetration" can fathom the life, for instance, of yonder mysterious, almost voiceless, Humming-Bird, smallest of feathery things, and loneliest, whirring among birds, insect-like, and among insects, bird-like, his path untraceable, his home unseen? An image of airy motion, yet it sometimes seems as if there were nothing joyous in him. He seems like some exiled pygmy prince, banished, but still regal, and doomed to wings. Did gems turn to flowers, flowers to feathers, in that long-past dynasty of the Humming-Birds? It is strange to come upon his tiny nest, in some gray and tangled swamp, with this brilliant atom perched disconsolately near it, upon some mossy twig; it is like visiting Cinderella among her ashes. And from Humming-Bird to Eagle, the daily existence of every bird is a remote and bewitching mystery.

Pythagoras has been charged, both before and since the days of Malvolio, with holding that "the soul of our grandam might haply inhabit a fowl,"—that delinquent men must revisit earth as women, and delinquent women as birds. Malvolio thought nobly of the soul, and in no way approved his opinion; but I remember that Harriet Rohan, in her school-days, accepted this, her destiny, with glee. "When I saw the Oriole," she wrote to me, "from his nest among the plum-trees in the garden, sail over the air and high above the Gothic arches of the elm, a stream of flashing light, or watched him swinging silently on pendent twigs, I did not dream how near akin we were. Or when a Humming-Bird, a winged drop of gorgeous sheen and gloss, a living gem, poising on his wings, thrust his dark, slender, honey-seeking bill into the white blossoms of a little bush beside my window, I should have thought it no such bad thing to be a bird, even if one next became a bat, like the colony in our eaves, that dart and drop and skim and skurry, all the length of moonless nights, in such ecstasies of dusky joy." Was this weird creature, the bat, in very truth a bird, in some far primeval time? and does he fancy, in unquiet dreams at nightfall, that he is one still? I wonder whether he can enjoy the winged brotherhood into which he has thrust himself, — victim, perhaps, of some rash quadruped-ambition, — an Icarus doomed forever *not* to fall.

I think, that, if required, on pain of death, to name instantly the most perfect thing in the universe, I should risk my fate on a bird's egg. There is, first, its exquisite fragility of material, strong only by the mathematical precision of that form so daintily moulded. There is its absolute purity from external stain, since that thin barrier remains impassable until the whole is in ruins, — a purity recognized in the household proverb of "An apple, an egg, and a nut." Then, its range of tints, so varied, so subdued, and so beautiful, — whether of pure white, like the Martin's, or pure green, like the Robin's, or dotted and mottled into the loveliest of browns, like the Red Thrush's, or aqua-marine, with stains of moss-agate, like the Chipping-Sparrow's, or blotched with long weird ink-marks on a pale ground, like the Oriole's, as if it bore inscribed some magic clew to the bird's darting flight and pensile nest. Above all, the associations and predictions of this little wonder, — that one may bear home between his fingers all that winged splendor, all that celestial melody, coiled in mystery within these tiny walls! Even the chrysalis is less amazing, for its form always preserves some trace, however fantastic, of the perfect insect, and it is but moulting a skin; but this egg appears to the eye like a separate unit from some other kingdom of Nature, claiming more kindred with the very stones than with feathery existence; and it is as if a pearl opened and an angel sang.

The nest which is to contain these fair things is a wondrous study also, from the coarse masonry of the Robin to the soft structure of the Humming-Bird, a baby-house among nests. Among all created things, the birds come nearest to man in their domesticity. Their unions are usually in pairs, and for life; and with them, unlike the practice of most quadrupeds, the male labors for the young. He chooses the locality of the nest, aids in its construction, and fights for it, if needful. He sometimes assists in hatching the eggs. He feeds the brood with exhausting labor, like yonder Robin, whose winged picturesque day is spent in putting worms into insatiable beaks, at the rate of one morsel in every three minutes. He has to teach them to fly, as among the Swallows, or even to hunt, as among the Hawks. His life is anchored to his home. Yonder Oriole fills with light and melody the thousand branches of a neighborhood; and yet the centre for all this divergent splendor is always that one drooping dome upon one chosen tree. This he helped to build in May, confiscating cotton as if he were a Union provost-marshal, and singing many songs, with his mouth full of plunder; and there he watches over his household, all through the leafy June, perched often upon the airy cradle-edge, and swaying with it in the summer wind. And from this deep nest, after the pretty eggs are hatched, will he and his mate extract every fragment of the shell, leaving it, like all other nests, save those of birds of prey, clean and pure, when the young are flown.

This they do chiefly from an instinct of delicacy; since wood-birds are not wont to use the same nest a second time, even if they rear several broods in a season.

The subdued tints and notes which almost always mark the female sex, among birds, — unlike insects and human beings, of which the female is often more showy than the male, — seem designed to secure their safety while sitting on the nest, while the brighter colors and louder song of the male enable his domestic circle to detect his whereabouts more easily. It is commonly noticed, in the same way, that ground-birds have more neutral tints than those which build out of reach. With the aid of these advantages, it is astonishing how well these roving creatures keep their secrets, and what sharp eyes are needed to spy out their habitations, — while it always seems as if the empty last-year's nests were very plenty. Some, indeed, are very elaborately concealed, as of the Golden-Crowned Thrush, called, for this reason, the Oven-Bird, — the Meadow-Lark, with its burrowed gallery among the grass, — and the Kingfisher, which mines four feet into the earth. But most of the rarer nests would hardly be discovered, only that the maternal instinct seems sometimes so overloaded by Nature as to defeat itself, and the bird flies and chirps in agony, when she might pass unnoticed by keeping still. The most marked exception which I have noticed is the Red Thrush, which, in this respect, as in others, has the most high-bred manners among all our birds: both male and female sometimes flit in perfect silence through the bushes, and show solicitude only in a sob which is scarcely audible.

Passing along the shore-path by our lake, one day in June, I heard a great sound of scuffling and yelping before me, as if dogs were hunting rabbits or woodchucks. On approaching, I saw no sign of such disturbances, and presently a Partridge came running at me through the trees, with ruff and tail expanded, bill wide open, and hissing like a Goose, — then turned suddenly, and with ruff and tail furled, but with no pretence of lameness, scudded off through the woods in a circle, — then at me again fiercely, approaching within two yards, and spreading all her furbelows, to intimidate, as before, — then, taking in sail, went off again, always at the same rate of speed, yelping like an angry squirrel, squealing like a pig, occasionally clucking like a hen, and, in general, so filling the woods with bustle and disturbance that there seemed no room for anything else. Quite overawed by the display, I stood watching her for some time, then entered the underbrush, where the little invisible brood had been unceasingly piping, in their baby way. So motionless were they, that, for all their noise, I stood with my feet among them, for some minutes, without finding it possible to detect them. When found and taken from the ground, which they so closely resembled, they made no attempt to escape; but when replaced, they presently ran away fast, as if conscious that the first policy had failed, and that their mother had retreated. Such is the summer life of these little things; but come again in the fall, when the wild autumnal winds go marching through the woods, and a dozen pairs of strong wings will thrill like thunder through the arches of the trees, as the full-grown brood whirrs away around you.

Not only have we scarcely any species of birds which are thoroughly and unquestionably identical with European species, but there are certain general variations of habit. For instance, in regard to migration. This is, of course, a universal instinct, since even tropical birds migrate for short distances from the equator, so essential to their existence do these wanderings seem. But in New England, among birds as among men, the roving habit seems unusually strong, and abodes are shifted very rapidly. The whole number of species observed in Massachusetts is about the same as in England, — some three hundred in all. But of this number, in England, about a hundred habitually winter on the island, and half that number even in the Hebrides, some birds actually breeding in Scotland during January and February, incredible as it may seem. Their habits can, therefore, be observed through a long period of the year; while with us the bright army comes and encamps for a month or two and then vanishes. You must attend their dress-parades, while they last; for you will have but few opportunities, and their domestic life must commonly be studied during a few weeks of the season, or not at all.

Wonderful as the instinct of migration seems, it is not, perhaps, so altogether amazing in itself as in some of its attendant details. To a great extent, birds follow the opening foliage northward, and flee from its fading, south; they must keep near the food on which they live, and secure due shelter for their eggs. Our earliest visitors shrink from trusting the bare trees with their nests; the Song-Sparrow seeks the ground; the Blue-Bird finds a box or a hole somewhere; the Red-Wing haunts the marshy thickets, safer in spring than at any other season; and even the sociable Robin prefers a pine-tree to an apple-tree, if resolved to begin housekeeping prematurely. The movements of birds are chiefly timed by the advance of vegetation; and the thing most thoroughly surprising about them is not the general fact of the change of latitude, but their accuracy in hitting the precise locality. That the same Cat-Bird should find its way back, every spring, to almost the same branch of yonder larch-tree,— that is the thing astonishing to me. In England, a lame Redstart was observed in the same garden for sixteen successive years; and the astonishing precision of course which enables some birds of small size to fly from Australia to New-Zealand in a day — probably the longest single flight ever taken — is only a part of the same mysterious instinct of direction.

In comparing modes of flight, the most surprising, of course, is that of the Swallow tribe, remarkable not merely for its velocity, but for the amazing boldness and instantaneousness of the angles it makes; so that eminent European mechanicians have speculated in vain upon the methods used in its locomotion, and prizes have been offered, by mechanical exhibitions, to him who could best explain it. With impetuous dash, they sweep through our perilous streets, these wild hunters of the air, "so near, and yet so far"; they bathe flying, and flying they feed their young. In my immediate vicinity, the Chimney-Swallow is not now common, nor the Sand-Swallow; but the Cliff-Swallow, that strange emigrant from the Far West, the Barn-Swallow, and the white-breasted species, are abundant, together with the Purple Martin. I know no prettier sight than a bevy of these bright little creatures, met from a dozen different farm-houses to picnic at a wayside pool, splashing and fluttering, with their long wings expanded like butterflies, keeping poised by a constant hovering motion, just tilting upon their feet, which scarcely touch the moist ground. You will seldom see them actually perch on anything less airy than some telegraphic wire; but when they do alight, each will make chatter enough for a dozen, as if all the rushing hurry of the wings had passed into the tongue.

Between the swiftness of the Swallow and the stateliness of the birds of prey, the whole range of bird-motion seems included. The long wave of a Hawk's wings seems almost to send a slow vibration through the atmosphere, tolling upon the eye as yon distant bell upon the ear. I never was more impressed with the superior dignity of these soarings than in observing a bloodless contest in the air, last April. Standing beside a little grove, on a rocky hillside, I heard Crows cawing near by, and then a sound like great flies buzzing, which I really attributed, for a moment, to some early insect. Turning, I saw two Crows flapping their heavy wings among the trees, and observed that they were teasing a Hawk about as large as themselves, which was also on the wing. Presently all three had risen above the branches, and were circling higher and higher in a slow spiral. The Crows kept constantly swooping at their enemy, with the same angry buzz, one of the two taking decidedly the lead. They seldom struck at him with their beaks, but kept lumbering against him, and flapping him with their wings, as if in a fruitless effort to capsize him; while the Hawk kept carelessly eluding the assaults, now inclining on one side, now on the other, with a stately grace, never retaliating, but seeming rather to enjoy the novel amusement, as if it were a skirmish in balloons. During all this, indeed, he scarcely seemed once to wave his wings; yet he soared steadily aloft, till the Crows refused to follow, though already higher than I ever saw Crows before, dim against the fleecy sky; then the Hawk flew northward, but soon after he sailed over us once again, with loud, scornful *chirr*, and they only cawed, and left him undisturbed.

When we hear the tumult of music from these various artists of the air, it seems as if the symphony never could be analyzed into its different instruments. But with time and patience it is not so difficult; nor can we really enjoy the performance, so long as it is only a confused chorus to our ears. It is not merely the highest form of animal language, but, in strictness of etymology, the only form, if it be true, as is claimed, that no other animal employs its tongue, *lingua*, in producing sound. In the Middle Ages, the song of birds was called their Latin, as was any other foreign dialect. It was the old German superstition, that any one who should eat the heart of a bird would thenceforth comprehend its language; and one modern philologist of the same nation (Masius declares) has so far studied the sounds produced by domestic fowls as to announce a Goose-Lexicon. Dupont de Nemours asserted that he understood eleven words of the Pigeon language, the same number of that of Fowls, fourteen of the Cat tongue, twenty-two of that of Cattle, thirty of that of Dogs, and the Raven language he understood completely. But the ordinary observer seldom attains farther than to comprehend some of the cries of anxiety and fear around him, often so unlike the accustomed carol of the bird, — as the mew of the Cat-Bird, the lamb-like bleating of the Veery and his impatient *yeoick*, the *chaip* of the Meadow-Lark, the *towyee* of the Chewink, the petulant *psit* and *tsee* of the Red-Winged Blackbird, and the hoarse cooing of the Bobolink. And with some of our most familiar birds the variety of notes is so great as really to promise difficulties in the American department of the bird-lexicon. I have watched two Song-Sparrows, perched near each other, in whom the spy-glass could show not the slightest difference of mark ing, even in the characteristic stains upon the breast, who yet chanted to each other, for fifteen minutes, over and over, two elaborate songs which had nothing in common. I have observed a similar thing in two Wood-Sparrows, with their sweet, distinct, accelerating lay; nor can I find it stated that the difference is sexual. Who can claim to have heard the whole song of the Robin? Taking shelter from a shower beneath an oak-tree, the other day, I caught a few of the notes which one of those cheery creatures, who love to sing in wet weather, tossed down to me through the drops.

(Before noticing me,)	*chirrup, cheerup;*
(pausing in alarm, at my approach,)	*che, che, che;*
(broken presently by a thoughtful strain,)	*caw, caw;*
(then softer and more confiding,)	*see, see, see;*
(then the original note, in a whisper,)	*chirrup, cheerup;*
(often broken by a soft note,)	*see, wee;*
(and an odder one,)	*squeal;*
(and a mellow note,)	*tweedle.*

And all these were mingled with more complex combinations, and with half-imitations, as of the Blue-Bird, so that it seemed almost impossible to doubt that there was some specific meaning, to him and his peers, in this endless vocabulary. Yet other birds, as quick-witted as the Robins, possess but one or two chirping notes, to which they seem unable to give more than the very rudest variation of accent.

The controversy between the singing-birds of Europe and America has had various phases and influential disputants. Buffon easily convinced himself that our Thrushes had no songs, because the voices of all birds grew harsh in savage countries, such as he naturally held this continent to be. Audubon, on the other hand, relates that even in his childhood he was assured by his father that the American songsters were the best, though neither Americans nor Europeans could be convinced of it. MacGillivray, the Scottish naturalist, reports that Audubon himself, in conversation, arranged our vocalists in the following order: — first, the Mocking-Bird, as unrivalled; then, the Wood-Thrush, Cat-Bird, and Red Thrush; the Rose-Breasted, Pine, and Blue Grosbeak; the Orchard and Golden Oriole; the Tawny and Hermit Thrushes; several Finches, — Bachmann's, the White-Crowned, the Indigo, and the Nonpareil; and finally, the Bobolink.

Among those birds of this list which frequent Massachusetts, Audubon might well put the Wood-Thrush at the head. As I sat the other day in the deep woods beside a black brook which dropped from stone to stone beneath the shadow of our Rattlesnake Rocks, the air seemed at first as silent above me as the earth below. The buzz of summer sounds had not begun. Sometimes a bee hummed by with a long swift thrill like a chord of music; sometimes a breeze came resounding up the forest like an approaching locomotive, and then died utterly away. Then, at length, a Veery's delicious note rose in a fountain of liquid melody from beneath me; and when it was ended, the clear, calm, interrupted chant of the Wood-Thrush fell like solemn water-drops from some source above. I am acquainted with no sound in Nature so sweet, so elevated, so serene. Flutes and flageolets are Art's poor efforts to recall that softer sound. It is simple, and seems all prelude; but the music to which it is the overture belongs to other spheres. It might be the *Angelus* of some lost convent. It might be the meditation of some maiden-hermit, saying over to herself in solitude, with recurrent tuneful pauses, the only song she knows.

Beside this soliloquy of seraphs, the carol of the Veery seems a familiar and almost domestic thing; yet it is so charming that Audubon must have designed to include it among the Thrushes whose merits he proclaims.

But the range of musical perfection is a wide one; and if the standard of excellence be that wondrous brilliancy and variety of execution suggested by the Mocking-Bird, then the palm belongs, among our New-England songsters, to the Red Thrush, otherwise called the Mavis or Brown Thrasher. I have never heard the Mocking-Bird sing at liberty; and while the caged bird may surpass the Red Thrush in volume of voice and in quaintness of direct imitation, he gives me no such impression of depth and magnificence. I know not how to describe the voluble and fantastic notes which fall like pearls and diamonds from the beak of our Mavis, while his stately attitudes and high-born bearing are in full harmony with the song. I recall the steep, bare hillside, and the two great boulders which guard the lonely grove, where I first fully learned the wonder of this lay, as if I had met Saint Cecilia there. A thoroughly happy song, overflowing with life, it gives even its most familiar phrases an air of gracious condescension, as when some great violinist stoops to the "Carnival of Venice." The Red Thrush does not, however, consent to any parrot-like mimicry, though every note of wood or field — Oriole, Bobolink, Crow, Jay, Robin, Whippoorwill — appears to pass in veiled procession through the song.

Retain the execution of the Red Thrush, but hopelessly impair his organ, and you have the Cat-Bird. This accustomed visitor would seem a gifted vocalist, but for the inevitable comparison between his thinner note and the gushing melodies of the lordlier bird. Is it some hopeless consciousness of this disadvantage which leads him to pursue that peculiar habit of singing softly to himself very often, in a fancied seclusion? When other birds are cheerily out-of-doors, on some bright morning of May or June, one will often discover a solitary Cat-Bird sitting concealed in the middle of a dense bush, and twittering busily, in subdued rehearsal, the whole copious variety of his lay, practising trills and preparing half-imitations, which, at some other time, sitting on the topmost twig, he shall hilariously seem to improvise before all the world. Can it be that he is really in some slight disgrace with Nature, with that demi-mourning garb of his, — and that his feline cry of terror, which makes his opprobrium with boys, is part of some hidden doom decreed? No, the lovely color of the eggs which his companion watches on that laboriously builded staging of twigs shall vindicate this familiar companion from any suspicion of original sin. Indeed, it is well demonstrated by our American oölogist, Dr. Brewer, that the eggs of the Cat-Bird affiliate him with the Robin and the Wood-Thrush, all three being widely separated in this respect from the Red Thrush. The Red Thrush builds on the ground, and has mottled eggs; while the whole household establishment of the Wood-Thrush is scarcely distinguishable from that of the Robin, and the Cat-Bird differs chiefly in being more of a carpenter and less of a mason.

The Rose-Breasted Grosbeak, which Audubon places so high on his list of minstrels, comes annually to one region in this vicinity, but I am not sure of having heard it. The young Pine Grosbeaks come to our woods in winter, and have then but a subdued twitter. Every one knows the Bobolink; and almost all recognize the Oriole, by sight at least, even if unfamiliar with all the notes of his cheery and resounding song. The Red-Eyed Fly-catcher, heard even more constantly, is less generally identified by name; but his note sounds all day among the elms of our streets, and seems a sort of piano-adaptation, popularized for the million, of the rich notes of the Thrushes. He is not mentioned by Audubon among his favorites, and has no right to complain of the exclusion. Yet the birds which most endear summer are not necessarily the finest performers; and certainly there is none whose note I could spare less easily than the little Chipping-Sparrow, called hereabouts the Hair-Bird. To lie half awake on a warm morning in June, and hear that soft insect-like chirp draw in and out with long melodious pulsations, like the rising and falling of the human breath, condenses for my ear the whole luxury of summer. Later in the day, among the multiplicity of noises, the chirping becomes louder and more detached, losing that faint and dream-like thrill.

The bird-notes which have the most familiar fascination are perhaps simply those most intimately associated with other rural things. This applies especially to the earliest spring songsters. Listening to these delicious prophets upon some of those still and moist days which slip in between the rough winds of March, and fill our lives for a moment with anticipated delights, it has seemed to me that their varied notes were sent to symbolize all the different elements of spring association. The Blue-Bird seems to represent simply spring's faint, tremulous, liquid sweetness, the Song-Sparrow its changing pulsations of more positive and varied joy, and the Robin its cheery and superabundant vitality. The later birds of the season, suggesting no such fine-drawn sensations, yet identify themselves with their chosen haunts, so that we cannot think of the one without the other. In the meadows, we hear the languid and tender drawl of the Meadow-Lark, — one of the most peculiar of notes, almost amounting to affectation in its excess of laborious sweetness. When we reach the thickets and wooded streams, there is no affectation in the Maryland Yellow-Throat, that little restless busybody, with his eternal *which-is-it, which-is-it, which-is-it,* emphasizing each syllable at will, in despair of response. Passing into the loftier woods, we find them resounding with the loud proclamation of the Golden-Crowned Thrush, — *scheat, scheat, scheat, scheat,* — rising and growing louder in a vigorous way that rather suggests some great Woodpecker than such a tiny thing. And penetrating to some yet lonelier place, we find it consecrated to that life-long sorrow, whatever it may be, which is made immortal in the plaintive cadence of the Pewee.

There is one favorite bird, — the Chewink, or Ground-Robin, — which, I always fancied, must have been known to Keats when he wrote those few words of perfect descriptiveness, —

> "If an innocent bird
> Before my heedless footsteps *stirred and stirred*
> *In little journeys.*"

What restless spirit is in this creature, that, while so shy in its own personal habits, it yet watches every visitor with a Paul-Pry curiosity, follows him in the woods, peers out among the underbrush, scratches upon the leaves with a pretty pretence of important business there, and presently, when disregarded, ascends some small tree and begins to carol its monotonous song, as if there were no such thing as man in the universe? There is something irregular and fantastic in the coloring, also, of the Chewink: unlike the generality of ground-birds, it is a showy thing, with black, white, and bay intermingled, and it is one of the most unmistakable of all our feathery creatures, in its aspect and its ways.

Another of my favorites, perhaps from our sympathy as to localities, since we meet freely every summer at a favorite lake, is the King-Bird or Tyrant-Flycatcher. The habits of royalty or tyranny I have never been able to perceive, — only a democratic habit of resistance to tyrants; but this bird always impresses me as a perfectly well-dressed and well-mannered person, who amid a very talkative society prefers to listen, and shows his character by action only. So long as he sits silently on some stake or bush in the neighborhood of his family circle, you notice only his glossy black cap and the white feathers in his handsome tail; but let a Hawk or a Crow come near, and you find that he is something more than a mere lazy listener to the Bobolink: far up in the air, determined to be thorough in his chastisements, you will see him, with a comrade or two, driving the bulky intruder away into the distance, till you wonder how he ever expects to find his own way back again. He speaks with emphasis on these occasions, and then reverts, more sedately than ever, to his accustomed silence.

After all the great labors of Audubon and Wilson, it is certain that the recent visible progress of American ornithology has by no means equalled that of several other departments of Natural History. The older books are now out of print, and there is actually no popular treatise on the subject to be had: a destitution singularly contrasted with the variety of excellent botanical works which the last twenty years have produced. Nuttall's fascinating volumes, and Brewer's edition of Wilson, are equally inaccessible; and the most valuable contributions since their time, so far as I know, are that portion of Dr. Brewer's work on eggs printed in the eleventh volume of the "Smithsonian Contributions," and four admirable articles in the Atlantic Monthly.* But the most important observations are locked up in the desks or exhibited in the cabinets of private observers, who have little opportunity of comparing facts with other students, or with reliable printed authorities. What do we know, for in stance, of the local distribution of our birds? I remember that in my latest conversation with Thoreau, last December, he mentioned most remarkable facts in this department, which had fallen under his unerring eyes. The Hawk most common at Concord, the Red-Tailed species, is not known near the sea-shore, twenty miles off, — as at Boston or Plymouth. The White-Breasted Sparrow is rare in Concord; but the Ashburnham woods, thirty miles away, are full of it. The Scarlet Tanager's is the commonest note in Concord, except the Red-Eyed Flycatcher's; yet one of the best field-ornithologists in Boston had never heard it. The Rose-Breasted Grosbeak is seen not infrequently at Concord, though its nest is rarely found; but in Minnesota Thoreau found it more abundant than any other bird, far more so than the Robin. But his most interesting statement, to my fancy, was, that, during a stay of ten weeks on Monadnock, he found that the Snow-Bird built its nest on the top of the mountain, and probably never came down through the season. That was its Arctic; and it would probably yet be found, he

* "Our Birds and their Ways" (December, 1857); "The Singing-Birds and their Songs" (August, 1858); "The Birds of the Garden and Orchard" (October, 1858); "The Birds of the Pasture and Forest" (December, 1858); — the first by J. Elliot Cabot, and the last three by Wilson Flagg.

predicted, on Wachusett and other Massachusetts peaks. It is known that the Snow-Bird, or "Snow-Flake," as it is called in England, was reported by Audubon as having only once been proved to build in the United States, namely, among the White Mountains, though Wilson found its nests among the Alleghanies; and in New England it used to be the rural belief that the Snow-Bird and the Chipping-Sparrow were the same.

After July, most of our birds grow silent, and, but for the insects, August would be almost the stillest month in the year, — stiller than the winter, when the woods are often vocal with the Crow, the Jay, and the Chickadee. But with patient attention one may hear, even far into the autumn, the accustomed notes. As I sat in my boat, one sunny afternoon of last September, beneath the shady western shore of our quiet lake, with the low sunlight striking almost level across the wooded banks, it seemed as if the last hoarded drops of summer's sweetness were being poured over all the world. The air was full of quiet sounds. Turtles rustled beside the brink and slid into the water, — cows plashed in the shallows, — fishes leaped from the placid depths, — a squirrel sobbed and fretted on a neighboring stump, — a katydid across the lake maintained its hard, dry croak, — the crickets chirped pertinaciously, but with little fatigued pauses, as if glad that their work was almost done, — the grasshoppers kept up their continual chant, which seemed thoroughly melted and amalgamated into the summer, as if it would go on indefinitely, though the body of the little creature were dried into dust. All this time the birds were silent and invisible, as if they would take no more part in the symphony of the year. Then, seemingly by preconcerted signal, they joined in: Crows cawed anxiously afar;

Jays screamed in the woods; a Partridge clucked to its brood, like the gurgle of water from a bottle; a Kingfisher wound his rattle, more briefly than in spring, as if we now knew all about it and the merest hint ought to suffice; a Fish-Hawk flapped into the water, with a great rude splash, and then flew heavily away; a flock of Wild Ducks went southward overhead, and a smaller party returned beneath them, flying low and anxiously, as if to pick up some lost baggage; and, at last, a Loon laughed loud from behind a distant island, and it was pleasant to people these woods and waters with that wild shouting, linking them with Katahdin Lake and Amperzand.

But the later the birds linger in the autumn, the more their aspect differs from that of spring. In spring, they come, jubilant, noisy, triumphant, from the South, the winter conquered and the long journey done. In autumn, they come timidly from the North, and, pausing on their anxious retreat, lurk within the fading copses and twitter snatches of song as fading. Others fly as openly as ever, but gather in flocks, as the Robins, most piteous of all birds at this season, — thin, faded, ragged, their bold note sunk to a feeble quaver, and their manner a mere caricature of that inexpressible military smartness with which they held up their heads in May.

Yet I cannot really find anything sad even in November. When I think of the thrilling beauty of the season past, the birds that came and went, the insects that took up the choral song as the birds grew silent, the procession of the flowers, the glory of autumn, — and when I think that, this also ended, a new gallery of wonder is opening, almost more beautiful, in the magnificence of frost and snow, — there comes an impression of affluence and liberality in the universe which seasons of changeless and uneventful verdure would never give. The catkins already formed on the alder, quite prepared to droop into April's beauty, — the white edges of the May-flower's petals, already visible through the bud, show in advance that winter is but a slight and temporary retardation of the life of Nature, and that the barrier which separates November from March is not really more solid than that which parts the sunset from the sunrise.

THE

PROCESSION OF THE FLOWERS.

THE PROCESSION OF THE FLOWERS.

IN Cuba there is a blossoming shrub whose multitudinous crimson flowers are so seductive to the humming-birds that they hover all day around it, buried in its blossoms until petal and wing seem one. At first upright, the gorgeous bells droop downward, and fall unwithered to the ground, and are thence called by the Creoles "Cupid's Tears." Fredrika Bremer relates that daily she brought home handfuls of these blossoms to her chamber, and nightly they all disappeared. One morning she looked toward the wall of the apartment, and there, in a long crimson line, the delicate flowers went ascending one by one to the ceiling, and passed from sight. She found that each was borne laboriously onward by a little colorless ant much smaller than itself: the bearer was invisible, but the lovely burdens festooned the wall with beauty.

To a watcher from the sky, the march of the flowers of any zone across the year would seem as beautiful as that West-Indian pageant. These frail creatures, rooted where they stand, a part of the "still life" of Nature, yet share her ceaseless motion. In the most sultry silence of summer noons, the vital current is coursing with desperate speed through the innumerable veins of every leaflet;

and the apparent stillness, like the sleeping of a child's top, is in truth the very ecstasy of perfected motion.

Not in the tropics only, but even in England, whence most of our floral associations and traditions come, the march of the flowers is in an endless circle, and, unlike our experience, something is always in bloom. In the Northern United States, it is said, the active growth of most plants is condensed into ten weeks, while in the mother country the full activity is maintained through sixteen. But even the English winter does not seem to be a winter, in the same sense as ours, appearing more like a chilly and comfortless autumn. There is no month in the year when some special plant does not bloom: the Coltsfoot there opens its fragrant flowers from December to February; the yellow-flowered Hellebore, and its cousin, the sacred Christmas Rose of Glastonbury, extend from January to March; and the Snowdrop and Primrose often come before the first of February. Something may be gained, much lost, by that perennial succession; those links, however slight, must make the floral period continuous to the imagination; while our year gives a pause and an interval to its children, and after exhausted October has effloresced into Witch-Hazel, there is an absolute reserve of blossom, until the Alders wave again.

No symbol could so well represent Nature's first yielding in spring-time as this blossoming of the Alder, this drooping of the tresses of these tender things. Before the frost is gone, and while the new-born season is yet too weak to assert itself by actually uplifting anything, it can at least let fall these blossoms, one by one, till they wave defiance to the winter on a thousand boughs. How patiently they have waited! Men are perplexed with anxieties about their own immortality; but these catkins, which hang, almost full-formed, above the ice all winter, show no such solicitude, but when March wooes them they are ready. Once relaxing, their pollen is so prompt to fall that it sprinkles your hand as you gather them; then, for one day, they are the perfection of grace upon your table, and next day they are weary and emaciated, and their little contribution to the spring is done.

Then many eyes watch for the opening of the May-flower, day by day, and a few for the Hepatica. So marked and fantastic are the local preferences of all our plants, that, with miles of woods and meadows open to their choice, each selects only some few spots for its accustomed abodes, and some one among them all for its very earliest blossoming. There is always some single chosen nook, which you might almost cover with your handkerchief, where each flower seems to bloom earliest, without variation, year by year. I know one such place for Hepatica a mile northeast, — another for May-flower two miles southwest; and each year the whimsical creature is in bloom on that little spot, when not another flower can be found open through the whole country round. Accidental as the choice may appear, it is undoubtedly based on laws more eternal than the stars; yet why all subtile influences conspire to bless that undistinguishable knoll no man can say. Another and similar puzzle offers itself in the distribution of the tints of flowers, — in these two species among the rest. There are certain localities, near by, where the Hepatica is all but white, and others where the May-flower is sumptuous in pink; yet it is not traceable to wet or dry, sun or shadow, and no agricultural chemistry can disclose the secret. Is it by some Darwinian law of selection that the white Hepatica has utterly overpowered the blue, in our Cascade Woods, for instance, while yet in the very midst of this pale plantation a single clump will sometimes bloom with all heaven on its petals? Why can one recognize the Plymouth May-flower, as soon as seen, by its wondrous depth of color? Does it blush with triumph to see how Nature has outwitted the Pilgrims, and even succeeded in preserving her deer like an English duke, still maintaining the deepest woods in Massachusetts precisely where those sturdy immigrants first began their clearings?

The Hepatica (called also Liverwort, Squirrel-Cup, or Blue Anemone) has been found in Worcester as early as March seventeenth, and in Danvers on March twelfth, — dates which appear almost the extreme of credibility.

Our next wild-flower in this region is the Claytonia, or Spring-Beauty, which is common in the Middle States, but here found in only a few localities. It is the Indian *Miskodeed*, and was said to have been left behind when mighty Peboan, the Winter, was melted by the breath of Spring. It is an exquisitely delicate little creature, bears its blossoms in clusters, unlike most of the early species, and opens in gradual succession each white and pink-veined bell. It grows in moist places on the sunny edges of woods, and prolongs its shy career from about the tenth of April until almost the end of May.

A week farther into April, and the Bloodroot opens, — a name of guilt, and a type of innocence. This fresh and lovely thing appears to concentrate all its stains within its ensanguined root, that it may condense all purity in the peculiar whiteness of its petals. It emerges from the ground with each shy blossom wrapt in its own pale-green leaf, then doffs the cloak and spreads its long petals round a group of yellow stamens. The flower falls apart so easily, that when in full bloom it will hardly bear transportation, but with a touch the stem stands naked, a bare gold-tipped sceptre amid drifts of snow. And the contradiction of its hues seems carried into its habits. One of the most shy of wild plants, easily banished from its locality by any invasion, it yet takes to the garden with unpardonable readiness, doubles its size, blossoms earlier, repudiates its love of water, and flaunts its great leaves in the unnatural confinement, until it elbows out the exotics. Its charm is gone, unless one find it in its native haunts, beside some cascade which streams over rocks that are dark with moisture, green with moss, and snowy with white bubbles. Each spray of dripping feather-moss exudes a tiny torrent of its own, or braided with some tiny neighbor, above the little water-fonts which sleep sunless in ever-verdant caves. Sometimes along these emerald canals there comes a sudden rush and hurry, as if some anxious housekeeper upon the hill above were afraid that things were not stirring fast enough,—and then again the waving and sinuous lines of water are quieted to a serener flow. The delicious red thrush and the busy little yellow-throat are not yet come to this their summer haunt; but all day long the answering field-sparrows trill out their sweet, shy, accelerating lay.

In the same localities with the Bloodroot, though some days later, grows the Dog-Tooth Violet,—a name hopelessly inappropriate, but likely never to be changed. These hardy and prolific creatures have also many localities of their own; for, though they do not acquiesce in cultivation, like the sycophantic Bloodroot, yet they are hard to banish from their native haunts, but linger after the woods are cleared and the meadow drained. The bright flowers blaze back all the yellow light of noonday, as the gay petals curl and spread themselves above their beds of mottled leaves; but it is always a disappointment to gather them, for in-doors they miss the full ardor of the sunbeams, and are apt to go to sleep and nod expressionless from the stalk.

And almost on the same day with this bright apparition one may greet a multitude of concurrent visitors, arriving so accurately together that it is almost a matter of accident which of the party shall first report himself. Perhaps the Dandelion should have the earliest place; indeed, I once found it in Brookline on the seventh of April. But it cannot ordinarily be expected before the twentieth, in Eastern Massachusetts, and rather later in the interior; while by the same date I have also found near Boston the Cowslip or Marsh-Marigold, the Spring-Saxifrage, the Anemones, the Violets, the Bellwort, the Houstonia, the Cinquefoil, and the Strawberry-blossom. Varying, of course, in different spots and years, the arrival of this coterie is yet nearly simultaneous, and they may all be expected hereabouts before May-day at the very latest. After all, in spite of the croakers, this festival could not have been much better timed, the delicate blossoms which mark the period are usually in perfection on this day, and it is not long before they are past their prime.

Some early plants which have now almost disappeared from Eastern Massachusetts are still found near Worcester in the greatest abundance, — as the larger Yellow Violet, the Red Trillium, the Dwarf Ginseng, the Clintonia or Wild Lily-of-the-Valley, and the pretty fringed Polygala, which Miss Cooper christened "Gay-Wings." Others again are now rare in this vicinity, and growing rarer, though still abundant a hundred miles farther inland. In several bits of old swampy wood one may still find, usually close together, the Hobble-Bush and the

Painted Trillium, the Mitella, or Bishop's-Cap, and the snowy Tiarella. Others again have entirely vanished within ten years, and that in some cases without any adequate explanation. The dainty white Corydalis, profanely called "Dutchman's Breeches," and the quaint woolly Ledum, or Labrador Tea, have disappeared within that time. The beautiful Linnæa is still found annually, but flowers no more; as is also the case, in all but one distant locality, with the once abundant Rhododendron. Nothing in Nature has for me a more fascinating interest than these secret movements of vegetation, — the sweet blind instinct with which flowers cling to old domains until absolutely compelled to forsake them. How touching is the fact, now well known, that salt-water plants still flower beside the Great Lakes, yet dreaming of the time when those waters were briny as the sea! Nothing in the demonstrations of Geology seems grander than the light lately thrown by Professor Gray, from the analogies between the flora of Japan and of North America, upon the successive epochs of heat which led the wandering flowers along the Arctic lands, and of cold which isolated them once more. Yet doubtless these humble movements of our local plants may be laying up results as important, and may hereafter supply evidence of earth's changes upon some smaller scale.

May expands to its prime of beauty; the summer birds come with the fruit-blossoms, the gardens are deluged with bloom, and the air with melody, while in the woods the timid spring flowers fold themselves away in silence and give place to a brighter splendor. On the margin of some quiet swamp a myriad of bare twigs seem suddenly overspread with purple butterflies, and we know that the Rhodora is in bloom. Wordsworth never immortalized a flower more surely than Emerson this, and it needs no weaker words; there is nothing else in which the change from nakedness to beauty is so sudden, and when you bring home the great mass of blossoms they appear all ready to flutter away again from your hands and leave you disenchanted.

At the same time the beautiful Cornel-tree is in perfection; startling as a tree of the tropics, it flaunts its great flowers high up among the forest-branches, intermingling its long slender twigs with theirs, and garnishing them with alien blooms. It is very available for household decoration, with its four great creamy petals, — flowers they are not, but floral involucres, — each with a fantastic curl and stain at its tip, as if the fire-flies had alighted on them and scorched them; and yet I like it best as it peers out in barbaric splendor from the delicate green of young Maples. And beneath it grows often its more abundant kinsman, the Dwarf Cornel, with the same four great petals enveloping its floral cluster, but lingering low upon the ground, — an herb whose blossoms mimic the statelier tree.

The same rich creamy hue and texture show themselves in the Wild Calla, which grows at this season in dark, sequestered water-courses, and sometimes well rivals, in all but size, that superb whiteness out of a land of darkness, the Ethiopic Calla of the conservatory. At this season, too, we seek another semi-aquatic rarity, whose homely name cannot deprive it of a certain garden-like elegance, the Buckbean. This is one of the shy plants which yet grow in profusion within their own domain. I have found it of old in Cambridge, and then upon the pleasant shallows of the Artichoke, that loveliest tributary of the Merrimack, and I have never seen it where it occupied a patch more than a few yards square, while yet within that space the multitudinous spikes grow always tall and close, reminding one of hyacinths, when in perfection, but more delicate and beautiful. The only locality I know for it in this vicinity lies seven miles away, where a little inlet from the lower winding bays of Lake Quinsigamond goes stealing up among a farmer's hay-fields, and there, close beside the public road and in full view of the farm-house, this rare creature fills the water. But to reach it we commonly row down the lake to a sheltered lagoon, separated from the main lake by a long island which is gradually forming itself like the coral isles, growing each year denser with alder thickets where the king-birds build; — there leave the boat among the lily-leaves, and take a lane which winds among the meadows and gives a fitting avenue for the pretty thing we seek. But it is not safe to vary many days from the twentieth of May, for the plant is not long in perfection, and is past its prime when the lower blossoms begin to wither on the stem.

But should we miss this delicate adjustment of time, it is easy to console ourselves with bright armfuls of Lupine, which bounteously flowers for six weeks along our lake-side, ranging from the twenty-third of May to the sixth of July. The Lupine is one of our most travelled plants; for, though never seen off the American continent, it stretches to the Pacific, and is found upon the Arctic coast. On these banks of Lake Quinsigamond it grows in great families, and should be gathered in masses and placed in a vase by itself; for it needs no relief from other flowers, its own soft leaves afford background enough, and though the white variety rarely occurs, yet the varying tints of blue upon the same stalk are a perpetual gratification to the eye. I know not why shaded blues should be so beautiful in flowers, and yet avoided as distasteful in ladies' fancy-work; but it is a mystery like that which repudiates blue-and-green from all well-regulated costumes, while Nature yet evidently prefers it to any other combination in her wardrobe.

Another constant ornament of the end of May is the large pink Lady's-Slipper, or Moccason-Flower, the "Cypripedium not due till to-morrow" which Emerson attributes to the note-book of Thoreau, — to-morrow, in these parts, meaning about the twentieth of May. It belongs to the family of Orchids, a high-bred race, fastidious in habits, sensitive as to abodes. Of the ten species named as rarest among American endogenous plants by Dr. Gray, in his valuable essay on the statistics of our Northern Flora, all but one are Orchids. And even an abundant species, like the present, retains the family traits in its person, and never loses its high-born air and its delicate veining. I know a grove where it can be gathered by the hundreds within a half-acre, and yet I never can divest myself of the feeling that each specimen is a choice novelty. But the actual rarity occurs, at least in this region, when one finds the smaller and more beautiful Yellow Moccason-Flower, — *parviflorum*, — which accepts only our very choicest botanical locality, the "Rattlesnake Ledge" on Tatessit Hill, — and may, for aught I know, have been the very plant which Elsie Venner laid upon her schoolmistress's desk.

June is an intermediate month between the spring and summer flowers. Of the more delicate early blossoms, the Dwarf Cornel, the Solomon's-Seal, and the Yellow Violet still linger in the woods, but rapidly make way for larger masses and more conspicuous hues. The meadows are gorgeous with Clover, Buttercups, and Wild Geranium; but Nature is a little chary for a week or two, maturing a more abundant show. Meanwhile one may afford to take some pains to search for another rarity, almost disappearing from this region, — the lovely Pink Azalea. It still grows plentifully in a few sequestered places, selecting woody swamps to hide itself; and certainly no shrub suggests, when found, more tropical associations. Those great, nodding, airy, fragrant clusters, tossing far above one's head their slender cups of honey, seem scarcely to belong to our sober zone, any more than the scarlet tanager which sometimes builds its nest beside them. They appear bright exotics, which have wandered into our woods, and seem too happy to feel any wish for exit. And just as they fade, their humbler sister in white begins to bloom, and carries on through the summer the same intoxicating fragrance.

But when June is at its height, the sculptured chalices of the Mountain Laurel begin to unfold, and thenceforward, for more than a month, extends the reign of this our woodland queen. I know not why one should sigh after the blossoming gorges of the Himalaya, when our forests are all so crowded with this glowing magnificence, — rounding the tangled swamps into smoothness, lighting up the underwoods, overtopping the pastures, lining the rural lanes, and rearing its great pinkish masses till they meet overhead. The color ranges from the purest white to a perfect rose-pink, and there is an inexhaustible vegetable vigor about the whole thing, which puts to shame those tenderer shrubs that shrink before the progress of cultivation. There is the Rhododendron, for instance, a plant of the same natural family with the Laurel and the Azalea, and looking more robust and woody than either:

it once grew in many localities in this region, and still lingers in a few, without consenting either to die or to blossom, and there is only one remote place from which any one now brings into our streets those large luxuriant flowers, waving white above the dark green leaves, and bearing "just a dream of sunset on their edges, and just a breath from the green sea in their hearts." But the Laurel, on the other hand, maintains its ground, imperturbable and almost impassable, on every hillside, takes no hints, suspects no danger, and nothing but the most unmistakable onset from spade or axe can diminish its profusion. Gathering it on the most lavish scale seems only to serve as wholesome pruning; nor can I conceive that the Indians, who once ruled over this whole county from Wigwam Hill, could ever have found it more inconveniently abundant than now. We have perhaps no single spot where it grows in such perfect picturesqueness as at "The Laurels," on the Merrimack, just above Newburyport, — a whole hillside scooped out and the hollow piled solidly with flowers, the pines curving around it above, and the river encircling it below, on which your boat glides along, and you look up through glimmering arcades of bloom. But for the last half of June it monopolizes everything in the Worcester woods, — no one picks anything else; and it fades so slowly that I have found a perfect blossom on the last day of July.

At the same time with this royalty of the woods, the queen of the water ascends her throne, for a reign as undisputed and far more prolonged. The extremes of the Water-Lily in this vicinity, so far as I have known, are the eighteenth of June and the thirteenth of October, — a longer range than belongs to any other conspicuous wild-flower, unless we except the Dandelion and Houstonia. It is not only the most fascinating of all flowers to gather, but more available for decorative purposes than almost any other, if it can only be kept fresh. The best method for this purpose, I believe, is to cut the stalk very short before placing in the vase; then, at night, the lily will close and the stalk curl upward; — refresh them by changing the water, and in the morning the stalk will be straight and the flower open.

From this time forth Summer has it all her own way. After the first of July the yellow flowers begin to watch the yellow fire-flies; Hawkweeds, Loosestrifes, Primroses bloom, and the bushy Wild Indigo. The variety of hues increases; delicate purple Orchises bloom in their chosen haunts, and Wild Roses blush over hill and dale. On peat-meadows the Adder's-Tongue Arethusa (now called *Pogonia*) flowers profusely, with a faint, delicious perfume, — and its more elegant cousin, the Calopogon, by its side. In this vicinity we miss the blue Harebell, the identical harebell of Ellen Douglas, which I remember waving its exquisite flowers along the banks of the Merrimack, and again at Brattleboro', below the cascade in the village, where it has climbed the precipitous sides of old buildings, and nods inaccessibly from their crevices, in that picturesque spot, looking down on the hurrying river. But with this exception, there is nothing wanting here of the flowers of early summer.

The more closely one studies Nature, the finer her adaptations grow. For instance, the change of seasons is analogous to a change of zones, and summer assimilates our vegetation to that of the tropics. In those lands, Humboldt has remarked, one misses the beauty of wild-flowers in the grass, because the luxuriance of vegetation develops everything into shrubs. The form and color are beautiful, "but, being too high above the soil, they disturb that harmonious proportion which characterizes the plants of our European meadows. Nature has, in every zone, stamped on the landscape the peculiar type of beauty proper to the locality." But every midsummer reveals the same tendency. In early spring, when all is bare, and small objects are easily made prominent, the wild-flowers are generally delicate. Later, when all verdure is profusely expanded, these miniature strokes would be lost, and Nature then practises landscape-gardening in large, lights up the copses with great masses of White Alder, makes the roadsides gay with Aster and Golden-Rod, and tops the tall coarse Meadow-Grass with nodding Lilies and tufted Spiræa. One instinctively follows these plain hints, and gathers bouquets sparingly in spring and exuberantly in summer.

The use of wild-flowers for decorative purposes merits a word in passing, for it is unquestionably a branch of high art in favored hands. It is true that we are bidden, on high authority, to love the wood-rose and leave it on its stalk; but against this may be set the saying of Bettine, that "all flowers which are broken become immortal in the sacrifice"; and certainly the secret harmonies of these fair creatures are so marked and delicate that we do not understand them till we try to group floral decorations for ourselves. The most successful artists will not, for instance, consent to put those together which do not grow together; Nature understands her business, and distributes her masses and backgrounds unerringly. Yonder soft and feathery Meadow-Sweet longs to be combined with Wild Roses: it yearns towards them in the field, and, after withering in the hand most readily, it revives in water as if to be with them in the vase. In the same way the White

Spiræa serves as natural background for the Field-Lilies. These lilies, by the way, are the brightest adornment of our meadows during the short period of their perfection. We have two species: one slender, erect, solitary, scarlet, looking up to heaven with all its blushes on; the other clustered, drooping, pale-yellow. I never saw the former in such profusion as last week, on the bare summit of Wachusett. The granite ribs have there a thin covering of crispest moss, spangled with the white starry blossoms of the Mountain Cinquefoil; and as I lay and watched the red lilies that waved their innumerable urns around me, it needed but little imagination to see a thousand altars, sending visible flames forever upward to the answering sun.

August comes: the Thistles are out, beloved of butterflies; deeper and deeper tints, more passionate intensities of color, prepare the way for the year's decline. A wealth of gorgeous Golden-Rod waves over all the hills, and enriches every bouquet one gathers; its bright colors command the eye, and it is graceful as an elm. Fitly arranged, it gives a bright relief to the superb beauty of the Cardinal-Flowers, the brilliant blue-purple of the Vervain, the pearl-white of the Life-Everlasting, the delicate lilac of the Monkey-Flower, the soft pink and white of the Spiræas, — for the white yet lingers, — all surrounded by trailing wreaths of blossoming Clematis.

But the Cardinal-Flower is best seen by itself, and, indeed, needs the surroundings of its native haunts to display its fullest beauty. Its favorite abode is along the dank mossy stones of some black and winding brook, shaded with overarching bushes, and running one long stream of scarlet with these superb occupants. It seems amazing how anything so brilliant can mature in such a darkness. When a ray of sunlight strays in upon it, the wondrous creature seems to hover on the stalk, ready to take flight, like some lost tropic bird. There is a spot whence I have in ten minutes brought away as many as I could hold in both arms, some bearing fifty blossoms on a single stalk; and I could not believe that there was such another mass of color in the world. Nothing cultivated is comparable to them; and, with all the talent lately lavished on wild-flower painting, I have never seen the peculiar sheen of these petals in the least degree delineated. It seems some new and separate tint, equally distinct from scarlet and from crimson, a splendor for which there is as yet no name, but only the reality.

It seems the signal of autumn, when September exhibits the first Barrel-Gentian by the roadside; and there is a pretty insect in the meadows — the Mourning-Cloak Moth it might be called — which gives coincident warning. The innumerable Asters mark this period with their varied and wide-spread beauty; the meadows are full of rose-colored Polygala, of the white spiral spikes of the Ladies'-Tresses, and of the fringed loveliness of the Gentian. This flower, always unique and beautiful, opening its delicate eyelashes every morning to the sunlight, closing them again each night, has also a thoughtful charm about it as the last of the year's especial darlings. It lingers long, each remaining blossom growing larger and more deep in color, as with many other flowers; and after it there is nothing for which to look forward, save the fantastic Witch-Hazel.

On the water, meanwhile, the last White Lilies are sinking beneath the surface, the last gay Pickerel-Weed is gone, though the rootless plants of the delicate Bladder-Wort, spreading over acres of shallows, still impurple the wide, smooth surface. Harriet Prescott says that some souls are like the Water-Lilies, fixed, yet floating. But others are like this graceful purple blossom, floating unfixed, kept in place only by its fellows around it, until perhaps a breeze comes, and, breaking the accidental cohesion, sweeps them all away.

The season reluctantly yields its reign, and over the quiet autumnal landscape everywhere, even after the glory of the trees is past, there are tints and fascinations of minor beauty. Last October, for instance, in walking, I found myself on a little knoll, looking northward. Overhead was a bower of climbing Waxwork, with its yellowish pods scarce disclosing their scarlet berries, — a wild Grape-vine, with its fruit withered by the frost into still purple raisins, — and yellow Beech-leaves, detaching themselves with an effort audible to the ear. In the foreground were blue Raspberry-stems, yet bearing greenish leaves, — pale-yellow Witch-Hazel, almost leafless, — purple Viburnum-berries, — the silky cocoons of the Milkweed, — and, amid the underbrush, a few lingering Asters and Golden-Rods, Ferns still green, and Maidenhair bleached white. In the background were hazy hills, white Birches bare and snow-like, and a Maple half-way up a sheltered hillside, one mass of canary-color, its fallen leaves making an apparent reflection on the earth at its foot, — and then a real reflection, fused into a glassy light intenser than itself, upon the smooth, dark stream below.

The beautiful disrobing suggested the persistent and unconquerable delicacy of Nature, who shrinks from nakedness and is always seeking to veil her graceful boughs, — if not with leaves, then with feathery hoarfrost, ermined snow, or transparent icy armor.

But, after all, the fascination of summer lies not in any

details, however perfect, but in the sense of total wealth which summer gives. Wholly to enjoy this, one must give one's self passively to it, and not expect to reproduce it in words. We strive to picture heaven, when we are barely at the threshold of the inconceivable beauty of earth. Perhaps the truant boy who simply bathes himself in the lake and then basks in the sunshine, dimly conscious of the exquisite loveliness around him, is wiser, because humbler, than is he who with presumptuous phrases tries to utter it. There are multitudes of moments when the atmosphere is so surcharged with luxury that every pore of the body becomes an ample gate for sensation to flow in, and one has simply to sit still and be filled. In after years the memory of books seems barren or vanishing, compared with the immortal bequest of hours like these. Other sources of illumination seem cisterns only; these are fountains. They may not increase the mere quantity of available thought, but they impart to it a quality which is priceless. No man can measure what a single hour with Nature may have contributed to the moulding of his mind. The influence is self-renewing, and if for a long time it baffles expression by reason of its fineness, so much the better in the end.

The soul is like a musical instrument: it is not enough that it be framed for the very most delicate vibration, but it must vibrate long and often before the fibres grow mellow to the finest waves of sympathy. I perceive that in the veery's carolling, the clover's scent, the glistening of the water, the waving wings of butterflies, the sunset tints, the floating clouds, there are attainable infinitely more subtile modulations of delight than I can yet reach the sensibility to discriminate, much less describe. If, in the simple process of writing, one could physically impart to this page the fragrance of this spray of azalea beside me, what a wonder would it seem! — and yet one ought to be able, by the mere use of language, to supply to every reader the total of that white, honeyed, trailing sweetness, which summer insects haunt and the Spirit of the Universe loves. The defect is not in language, but in men. There is no conceivable beauty of blossom so beautiful as words, — none so graceful, none so perfumed. It is possible to dream of combinations of syllables so delicious that all the dawning and decay of summer cannot rival their perfection, nor winter's stainless white and azure match their purity and their charm. To write them, were it possible, would be to take rank with Nature; nor is there any other method, even by music, for human art to reach so high.

SNOW.

SNOW.

ALL through the long hours of yesterday the low clouds hung close above our heads, to pour with more unswerving aim their constant storm of sleet and snow, — sometimes working in soft silence, sometimes with impatient gusty breaths, but always busily at work. Darkness brought no rest to these laborious warriors of the air, but only fiercer strife: the wild winds rose; noisy recruits, they howled beneath the eaves, or swept around the walls, like hungry wolves, now here, now there, howling at opposite doors. Thus, through the anxious and wakeful night, the storm went on. The household lay vexed by broken dreams, with changing fancies of lost children on solitary moors, of sleighs hopelessly overturned in drifted and pathless gorges, or of icy cordage upon disabled vessels in Arctic seas; until a softer warmth, as of sheltering snow-wreaths, lulled all into deeper rest till morning.

And what a morning! The sun, a young conqueror, sends in his glorious rays, like heralds, to rouse us for the inspection of his trophies. The baffled foe, retiring, has left far and near the high-heaped spoils behind. The glittering plains own the new victor. Over all these level and wide-swept meadows, over all these drifted, spotless slopes, he is proclaimed undisputed monarch. On the wooded hillsides the startled shadows are in motion; they flee like young fawns, bounding upward and downward over rock and dell, as through the long gleaming arches the king comes marching to his throne. But shade yet lingers undisturbed in the valleys, mingled with timid smoke from household chimneys; blue as the smoke, a gauzy haze is twined around the brow of every distant hill; and the same soft azure confuses the outlines of the nearer trees, to whose branches snowy wreaths are clinging, far up among the boughs, like strange new flowers. Everywhere the unstained surface glistens in the sunbeams. In the curves and wreaths and turrets of the drifts a blue tinge nestles. The fresh pure sky answers to it; every cloud has vanished, save one or two which linger near the horizon, pardoned offenders, seeming far too innocent for mischief, although their dark and sullen brothers, banished ignominiously below the horizon's verge, may be plotting nameless treachery there. The brook still flows visibly through the valley, and the myriad rocks that check its course are all rounded with fleecy surfaces, till they seem like flocks of tranquil sheep that drink the shallow flood.

The day is one of moderate cold, but clear and bracing; the air sparkles like the snow; everything seems dry and resonant, like the wood of a violin. All sounds are musical, — the voices of children, the cooing of doves, the crowing of cocks, the chopping of wood, the creaking of country sleds, the sweet jangle of sleigh-bells. The snow has fallen under a cold temperature, and the flakes are perfectly crystallized; every shrub we pass bears wreaths which glitter as gorgeously as the nebula in the constellation Perseus; but in another hour of sunshine every one of those fragile outlines will disappear, and the white surface glitter no longer with stars, but with star-dust. On such a day, the universe seems to hold but three pure tints, — blue, white, and green. The loveliness of the universe seems simplified to its last extreme of refined delicacy. That sensation we poor mortals often have, of being just on the edge of infinite beauty, yet with always a lingering film between, never presses down more closely than on days like this. Everything seems perfectly prepared to satiate the soul with inexpressible felicity, if we could only, by one infinitesimal step farther, reach the mood to dwell in it.

Leaving behind us the sleighs and snow-shovels of the street, we turn noiselessly toward the radiant margin of the sunlit woods. The yellow willows on the causeway burn like flame against the darker background, and will burn on until they burst into April. Yonder pines and hemlocks stand motionless and dark against the sky. The statelier trees have already shaken all the snow from their summits, but it still clothes the lower ones with a white covering that looks solid as marble. Yet see how lightly it escapes! — a slight gust shakes a single tree, there is a *Staub-bach* for a moment, and the branches stand free as in summer, a pyramid of green amid the whiteness of the yet imprisoned forest. Each branch raises itself when emancipated, thus changing the whole outline of the growth; and the snow beneath is punctured with a thousand little depressions, where the petty avalanches have just buried themselves and disappeared.

In crossing this white level, we have been tracking our way across an invisible pond, which was alive last week with five hundred skaters. Now there is a foot of snow upon it, through which there is a boyish excitement in making the first path. Looking back upon our track, it proves to be like all other human paths, straight in intention, but slightly devious in deed. We have gay companions on our way; for a breeze overtakes us, and a hundred little simooms of drift whirl along beside us, and whelm in miniature burial whole caravans of dry leaves. Here, too, our track intersects with that of some previous passer; he has but just gone on, judging by the freshness of the trail, and we can study his character and purposes. The large boots betoken a woodman or iceman; yet such a one would hardly have stepped so irresolutely where a little film of water has spread between the ice and snow and given a look of insecurity; and here again he has stopped to observe the wreaths on this pendent bough, and this snow-filled bird's-nest. And there the footsteps of the lover of beauty turn abruptly to the road again, and he vanishes from us forever.

As we wander on through the wood, all the labyrinths of summer are buried beneath one white inviting pathway, and the pledge of perfect loneliness is given by the unbroken surface of the all-revealing snow. There appears nothing living except a downy woodpecker, whirling round and round upon a young beech-stem, and a few sparrows, plump with grass-seed and hurrying with jerking flight down the sunny glade. But the trees furnish society enough. What a congress of ermined kings is this circle of hemlocks, which stand, white in their soft raiment, around the dais of this woodland pond! Are they held here, like the sovereigns in the palace of the Sleeping Beauty, till some mortal breaks their spell? What sage counsels must be theirs, as they nod their weary heads and whisper ghostly memories and old men's tales to each other, while the red leaves dance on the snowy sward below, or a fox or squirrel steals hurriedly through the wild and wintry night! Here and there is some discrowned Lear, who has thrown off his regal mantle, and stands in faded russet, misplaced among the monarchs.

What a simple and stately hospitality is that of Nature in winter! The season which the residents of cities think an obstruction is in the country an extension of intercourse: it opens every forest from here to Labrador, free of entrance; the most tangled thicket, the most treacherous marsh, becomes passable; and the lumberer or moose-hunter, mounted on his snow-shoes, has the world before him. He says "good snow-shoeing," as we say "good sleighing"; and it gives a sensation like a first visit to the sea-side and the shipping, when one first sees exhibited for sale, in the streets of Bangor or Montreal, these delicate Indian conveyances. It seems as if a new element were suddenly opened for travel, and all due facilities provided. One expects to go a little farther, and see in the shop-windows, "Wings for sale, — gentlemen's and ladies' sizes." The snow-shoe and the birch canoe, — what other dying race ever left behind it two memorials so perfect and so graceful.

The shadows thrown by the trees upon the snow are blue and soft, sharply defined, and so contrasted with the gleaming white as to appear narrower than the boughs which cast them. There is something subtle and fantastic about these shadows. Here is a leafless larch-sapling, eight feet high. The image of the lower boughs is traced upon the snow, distinct and firm as cordage, while the higher ones grow dimmer by fine gradations, until the slender topmost twig is blurred, and almost effaced. But the denser upper spire of the young spruce by its side throws almost as distinct a shadow as its base, and the whole figure looks of a more solid texture, as if you could feel it with your hand. More beautiful than either is the fine image of this baby hemlock: each delicate leaf droops above as delicate a copy, and here and there the shadow and the substance kiss and frolic with each other in the downy snow.

The larger larches have a different plaything: on the bare branches, thickly studded with buds, cling airily the small, light cones of last year's growth, each crowned with a little ball of soft snow, four times taller than itself, — save where some have drooped sideways, so that each carries, poor weary Atlas, a sphere upon its back. Thus the coy creatures play cup and ball, and one has lost its plaything yonder, as the branch slightly stirs, and the whole vanishes in a whirl of snow. Meanwhile a fragment of low arbor-vitæ hedge, poor outpost of a neighboring plantation, is so covered and packed with solid drift, inside and out, that it seems as if no power of sunshine could ever steal in among its twigs and disentangle it.

In winter each separate object interests us; in summer, the mass. Natural beauty in winter is a poor man's luxury, infinitely enhanced in quality by the diminution in quantity. Winter, with fewer and simpler methods, yet seems to give all her works a finish even more delicate than that of summer, working, as Emerson says of English agriculture, with a pencil, instead of a plough. Or rather, the ploughshare is but concealed; since a pithy old English preacher has said that "the frost is God's plough, which he drives through every inch of ground in the world, opening each clod, and pulverizing the whole."

Coming out upon a high hillside, more exposed to the

direct fury of the sleet, we find Nature wearing a wilder look. Every white-birch clump around us is bent divergingly to the ground, each white form prostrated in mute despair upon the whiter bank. The bare, writhing branches of yonder sombre oak-grove are steeped in snow, and in the misty air they look so remote and foreign that there is not a wild creature of the Norse mythology who might not stalk from beneath their haunted branches. Buried races, Teutons and Cimbri, might tramp solemnly forth from those weird arcades. The soft pines on this nearer knoll seem separated from them by ages and generations. On the farther hills spread woods of smaller growth, like forests of spun glass, jewelry by the acre provided for this coronation of winter.

We descend a steep bank, little pellets of snow rolling hastily beside us, and leaving enamelled furrows behind. Entering the sheltered and sunny glade, we are assailed by a sudden warmth whose languor is almost oppressive. Wherever the sun strikes upon the pines and hemlocks, there is a household gleam which gives a more vivid sensation than the diffused brilliancy of summer. The sunbeams maintain a thousand secondary fires in the reflection of light from every tree and stalk, for the preservation of animal life and ultimate melting of these accumulated drifts. Around each trunk or stone the snow has melted and fallen back. It is a singular fact, established beyond doubt by science, that the snow is absolutely less influenced by the direct rays of the sun than by these reflections. "If a blackened card is placed upon the snow or ice in the sunshine, the frozen mass underneath it will be gradually thawed, while that by which it is surrounded, though exposed to the full power of solar heat, is but little disturbed. If, however, we reflect the sun's rays from a metal surface, an exactly contrary result takes place: the uncovered parts are the first to melt, and the blackened card stands high above the surrounding portion." Look round upon this buried meadow, and you will see emerging through the white surface a thousand stalks of grass, sedge, osmunda, golden-rod, mullein, Saint-John's-wort, plaintain, and eupatorium, — an allied army of the sun, keeping up a perpetual volley of innumerable rays upon the yielding snow.

It is their last dying service. We misplace our tenderness in winter, and look with pity upon the leafless trees. But there is no tragedy in the trees: each is not dead, but sleepeth; and each bears a future summer of buds safe nestled on its bosom, as a mother reposes with her baby at her breast. The same security of life pervades every woody shrub: the alder and the birch have their catkins all ready for the first day of spring, and the sweet-fern has even now filled with fragrance its folded blossom. Winter is no such solid bar between season and season as we fancy, but only a slight check and interruption: one may at any time produce these March blossoms by bringing the buds into the warm house; and the petals of the May-flower sometimes show their pink and white edges in autumn. But every grass-blade and flower-stalk is a mausoleum of vanished summer, itself crumbling to dust, never to rise again. Each child of June, scarce distinguishable in November against the background of moss and rocks and bushes, is brought into final prominence in December by the white snow which imbeds it. The delicate flakes collapse and fall back around it, but retain their inexorable hold. Thus delicate is the action of Nature, — a finger of air, and a grasp of iron.

We pass the old red foundry, banked in with snow and

its low eaves draped with icicles, and come to the brook which turns its resounding wheel. The musical motion of the water seems almost unnatural amidst the general stillness: brooks, like men, must keep themselves warm by exercise. The overhanging rushes and alder-sprays, weary of winter's sameness, have made for themselves playthings, — each dangling a crystal knob of ice, which sways gently in the water and gleams ruddy in the sunlight. As we approach the foaming cascade, the toys become larger and more glittering, movable stalactites, which the water tosses merrily upon their flexible stems. The torrent pours down beneath an enamelled mask of ice, wreathed and convoluted like a brain, and sparkling with gorgeous glow. Tremulous motions and glimmerings go through the translucent veil, as if it throbbed with the throbbing wave beneath. It holds in its mazes stray bits of color, — scarlet berries, evergreen sprigs, blue raspberry-stems, and sprays of yellow willow; glittering necklaces and wreaths and tiaras of brilliant ice-work cling and trail around its edges, and no regal palace shines with such carcanets of jewels as this winter ball-room of the dancing drops.

Above, the brook becomes a smooth black canal between two steep white banks; and the glassy water seems momentarily stiffening into the solider blackness of ice. Here and there thin films are already formed over it, and are being constantly broken apart by the treacherous current; a flake a foot square is jerked away and goes sliding beneath the slight transparent surface till it reappears below. The same thing, on a larger scale, helps to form the mighty ice-pack of the Northern seas. Nothing except ice is capable of combining, on the largest scale, bulk with mobility, and this imparts a dignity to its motions even on the smallest scale. I do not believe that anything in Behring's Straits could impress me with a grander sense of desolation or of power, than when in boyhood I watched the ice break up in the winding channel of Charles River.

Amidst so much that seems like death, let us turn and study the life. There is much more to be seen in winter than most of us have ever noticed. Far in the North the "moose-yards" are crowded and trampled, at this season, and the wolf and the deer run noiselessly a deadly race, as I have heard the hunters describe, upon the white surface of the gleaming lake. But the pond beneath our feet keeps its stores of life chiefly below its level platform, as the bright fishes in the basket of yon heavy-booted fisherman can tell. Yet the scattered tracks of mink and muskrat beside the banks, of meadow-mice around the hay-stacks, of squirrels under the trees, of rabbits and partridges in the wood, show the warm life that is beating unseen, beneath fur or feathers, close beside us. The chickadees are chattering merrily in the upland grove, the blue-jays scream in the hemlock glade, the snow-bird mates the snow with its whiteness, and the robin contrasts with it his still ruddy breast. The weird and impenetrable crows, most talkative of birds and most uncommunicative, their very food at this season a mystery, are almost as numerous now as in summer. They always seem like some race of banished goblins, doing penance for some primeval and inscrutable transgression, and if any bird have a history, it is they. In the Spanish version of the tradition of King Arthur, it is said that he fled from the weeping queens and the island valley of Avilion in the form of a crow; and hence it is said in "Don Quixote" that no Englishman will ever kill one.

The traces of the insects in the winter are prophetic,—from the delicate cocoon of some infinitesimal feathery thing which hangs upon the dry, starry calyx of the aster, to the large brown-paper parcel which hides in peasant garb the costly beauty of some gorgeous moth. But the hints of birds are retrospective. In each tree of this pasture, the very pasture where last spring we looked for nests and found them not among the deceitful foliage, the fragile domiciles now stand revealed. But where are the birds that filled them? Could the airy creatures nurtured in those nests have left permanently traced upon the air behind them their own bright summer flight, the whole atmosphere would be filled with interlacing lines and curves of gorgeous coloring, the centre of all being this forsaken bird's-nest filled with snow.

Among the many birds which winter here, and the many insects which are called forth by a few days of thaw, not a few must die of cold or of fatigue amid the storms. Yet how few traces one sees of this mortality! Provision is made for it. Yonder a dead wasp has fallen on the snow, and the warmth of its body, or its power of reflecting a few small rays of light, is melting its little grave beneath it. With what a cleanly purity does Nature strive to withdraw all unsightly objects into her cemetery! Their own weight and lingering warmth take them through air or water, snow or ice, to the level of the earth, and there with spring comes an army of burying-insects, *Necrophagi*, in a livery of red and black, to dig a grave beneath every one, and not a sparrow falleth to the ground without knowledge. The tiny remains thus disappear from the surface, and the dry leaves are soon spread above these Children in the Wood.

Thus varied and benignant are the aspects of winter on

these sunny days. But it is impossible to claim this weather as the only type of our winter climate. There occasionally come days which, though perfectly still and serene, suggest more terror than any tempest, — terrible, clear, glaring days of pitiless cold, — when the sun seems powerless or only a brighter moon, when the windows remain ground-glass at high noontide, and when, on going out of doors, one is dazzled by the brightness, and fancies for a moment that it cannot be so cold as has been reported, but presently discovers that the severity is only more deadly for being so still. Exercise on such days seems to produce no warmth; one's limbs appear ready to break on any sudden motion, like icy boughs. Stage-drivers and draymen are transformed to mere human buffaloes by their fur coats; the patient oxen are frost-covered; the horse that goes racing by waves a wreath of steam from his tossing head. On such days life becomes a battle to all householders, the ordinary apparatus for defence is insufficient, and the price of caloric is continual vigilance. In innumerable armies the frost besieges the portal, creeps in beneath it and above it, and on every latch and key-handle lodges an advanced guard of white rime. Leave the door ajar never so slightly, and a chill creeps in cat-like; we are conscious by the warmest fireside of the near vicinity of cold, its fingers are feeling after us, and even if they do not clutch us, we know that they are there. The sensations of such days almost make us associate their clearness and whiteness with something malignant and evil. Charles Lamb asserts of snow, "It glares too much for an innocent color, methinks." Why does popular mythology associate the infernal regions with a high temperature instead of a low one? El Aishi, the Arab writer, says of the bleak wind of the Desert, (so writes Richardson, the African traveller,) "The north wind blows with an intensity equalling *the cold of hell;* language fails me to describe its rigorous temperature." Some have thought that there is a similar allusion in the phrase, "weeping and gnashing of teeth," — the teeth chattering from frost. Milton also enumerates cold as one of the torments of the lost, —

"O'er many a frozen, many a fiery Alp";

and one may sup full of horrors on the exceedingly cold collation provided for the next world by the Norse Edda.

But, after all, there are but few such terrific periods in our Massachusetts winters, and the appointed exit from their frigidity is usually through a snow-storm. After a day of this severe sunshine there comes commonly a darker day of cloud, still hard and forbidding, though milder in promise, with a sky of lead, deepening near the horizon into darker films of iron. Then, while all the nerves of the universe seem rigid and tense, the first reluctant flake steals slowly down, like a tear. In a few hours the whole atmosphere begins to relax once more, and in our astonishing climate very possibly the snow changes to rain in twenty-four hours, and a thaw sets in. It is not strange, therefore, that snow, which to Southern races is typical of cold and terror, brings associations of warmth and shelter to the children of the North.

Snow, indeed, actually nourishes animal life. It holds in its bosom numerous animalcules: you may have a glass of water, perfectly free from *infusoria,* which yet, after your dissolving in it a handful of snow, will show itself full of microscopic creatures, shrimp-like and swift; and the famous red snow of the Arctic regions is only an exhibition of the same property. It has sometimes been fancied that persons buried under the snow have received sustenance through the pores of the skin, like reptiles imbedded in rock. Elizabeth Woodcock lived eight days beneath a snow-drift, in 1799, without eating a morsel; and a Swiss family were buried beneath an avalanche, in a manger, for five months, in 1755, with no food but a trifling store of chestnuts and a small daily supply of milk from a goat which was buried with them. In neither case was there extreme suffering from cold, and it is unquestionable that the interior of a drift is far warmer than the surface. On the 23d of December, 1860, at 9 P. M., I was surprised to observe drops falling from the under side of a heavy bank of snow at the eaves, at a distance from any chimney, while the mercury on the same side was only fifteen degrees above zero, not having indeed risen above the point of freezing during the whole day.

Dr. Kane pays ample tribute to these kindly properties. "Few of us at home can recognize the protecting value of this warm coverlet of snow. No eider-down in the cradle of an infant is tucked in more kindly than the sleeping-dress of winter about this feeble flower-life. The first warm snows of August and September, falling on a thickly pleached carpet of grasses, heaths, and willows, enshrine the flowery growths which nestle round them in a non-conducting air-chamber; and as each successive snow increases the thickness of the cover, we have, before the intense cold of winter sets in, a light cellular bed covered by drift, six, eight, or ten feet deep, in which the plant retains its vitality. . . . . . I have found in midwinter, in this high latitude of 78° 50′, the surface so nearly moist as to be friable to the touch; and upon the ice-floes, commencing with a surface-temperature of

—30°, I found at two feet deep a temperature of —8°, at four feet +2°, and at eight feet +26°. . . . . The glacier which we became so familiar with afterwards at Etah yields an uninterrupted stream throughout the year." And he afterwards shows that even the varying texture and quality of the snow deposited during the earlier and later portions of the Arctic winter have their special adaptations to the welfare of the vegetation they protect.

The process of crystallization seems a microcosm of the universe. Radiata, mollusca, feathers, flowers, ferns, mosses, palms, pines, grain-fields, leaves of cedar, chestnut, elm, acanthus: these and multitudes of other objects are figured on your frosty window; on sixteen different panes I have counted sixteen patterns strikingly distinct, and it appeared like a show-case for the globe. What can seem remoter relatives than the star, the star-fish, the star-flower, and the starry snow-flake which clings this moment to your sleeve? — yet some philosophers hold that one day their law of existence will be found precisely the same. The connection with the primeval star, especially, seems far and fanciful enough, but there are yet unexplored affinities between light and crystallization: some crystals have a tendency to grow toward the light, and others develop electricity and give out flashes of light during their formation. Slight foundations for scientific fancies, indeed, but slight is all our knowledge.

More than a hundred different figures of snow-flakes, all regular and kaleidoscopic, have been drawn by Scoresby, Lowe, and Glaisher, and may be found pictured in the encyclopædias and elsewhere, ranging from the simplest stellar shapes to the most complicated ramifications. Professor Tyndall, in his delightful book on "The Glaciers of the Alps," gives drawings of a few of these snow-blossoms, which he watched falling for hours, the whole air being filled with them, and drifts of several inches being accumulated while he watched. "Let us imagine the eye gifted with microscopic power sufficient to enable it to see the molecules which composed these starry crystals; to observe the solid nucleus formed and floating in the air; to see it drawing towards it its allied atoms, and these arranging themselves as if they moved to music, and ended with rendering that music concrete." Thus do the Alpine winds, like Orpheus, build their walls by harmony.

In some of these frost-flowers the rare and delicate blossom of our wild *Mitella diphylla* is beautifully figured. Snow-flakes have been also found in the form of regular hexagons and other plane figures, as well as in cylinders and spheres. As a general rule, the intenser the cold the more perfect the formation, and the most perfect specimens are Arctic or Alpine in their locality. In this climate the snow seldom falls when the mercury is much below zero; but the slightest atmospheric changes may alter the whole condition of the deposit, and decide whether it shall sparkle like Italian marble, or be dead-white like the statuary marble of Vermont, — whether it shall be a fine powder which can sift through wherever dust can, or descend in large woolly masses, tossed like mouthfuls to the hungry earth.

The most remarkable display of crystallization which I have ever seen was on the 13th of January, 1859. There had been three days of unusual cold, but during the night the weather had moderated, and the mercury in the morning stood at $+14°$. About two inches of snow had fallen, and the trees appeared densely coated with it. It proved, on examination, that every twig had on the leeward side a dense row of miniature fronds or fern-leaves executed in snow, with a sharply defined central nerve, or midrib, and perfect ramification, tapering to a point, and varying in length from half an inch to three inches. On every post, every rail, and the corners of every building, the same spectacle was seen; and where the snow had accumulated in deep drifts, it was still made up of the ruins of these fairy structures. The white, enamelled landscape was beautiful, but a close view of the details was far more so. The crystallizations were somewhat uniform in structure, yet suggested a variety of natural objects, as feather-mosses, birds' feathers, and the most delicate lace-corals, but the predominant analogy was with ferns. Yet they seemed to assume a sort of fantastic kindred with the objects to which they adhered: thus, on the leaves of spruce-trees and on delicate lichens they seemed like reduplications of the original growth, and they made the broad, flat leaves of the arbor-vitæ fully twice as wide as before. But this fringe was always on one side only, except when gathered upon dangling fragments of spider's web, or bits of stray thread: these they entirely encircled, probably because these objects had twirled in the light wind while the crystals were forming. Singular disguises were produced: a bit of ragged rope appeared a piece of twisted lace-work; a knot-hole in a board was adorned with a deep antechamber of snowy wreaths; and the frozen body of a hairy caterpillar became its own well-plumed hearse. The most peculiar circumstance was the fact that single flakes never showed any regular crystallization: the magic was in the combination; the under sides of rails and boards exhibited it as unequivocally as the upper sides, indicating that the phenomenon was created in the lower atmosphere, and was more akin to frost than snow; and yet the largest snow-banks were composed of nothing else, and seemed like heaps of blanched iron-filings.

Interesting observations have been made on the relations between ice and snow. The difference seems to lie only in the more or less compacted arrangement of the frozen particles. Water and air, each being transparent when separate, become opaque when intimately mingled; the reason being that the inequalities of refraction break up and scatter every ray of light. Thus, clouds cast a shadow; so does steam; so does foam: and the same elements take a still denser texture when combined as snow. Every snow-flake is permeated with minute airy chambers, among which the light is bewildered and lost; while from perfectly hard and transparent ice every trace of air disappears, and the transmission of light is unbroken. Yet that same ice becomes white and opaque when pulverized, its fragments being then intermingled with air again,—just as colorless glass may be crushed into white powder. On the other hand, Professor Tyndall has converted slabs of snow to ice by regular pressure, and has shown that every Alpine glacier begins as a snow-drift at its summit, and ends in a transparent ice-cavern below. "The blue blocks which span the sources of the Arveiron were once powdery snow upon the slopes of the Col du Géant."

The varied and wonderful shapes assumed by snow and ice have been best portrayed, perhaps, by Dr. Kane in his two works; but their resources of color have been so explored by no one as by this same favored Professor Tyndall, among his Alps. It appears that the tints which in temperate regions are seen feebly and occasionally, in hollows or angles of fresh drifts, become brilliant and constant above the line of perpetual snow, and the higher the altitude the more lustrous the display. When a staff was struck into the new-fallen drift, the hollow seemed instantly to fill with a soft blue liquid, while the snow adhering to the staff took a complementary color of pinkish yellow, and on moving it up and down it was hard to resist the impression that a pink flame was rising and sinking in the hole. The little natural furrows in the drifts appeared faintly blue, the ridges were gray, while the parts most exposed to view seemed least illuminated, and as if a light brown dust had been sprinkled over them. The fresher the snow, the more marked the colors, and it made no difference whether the sky were cloudless or foggy. Thus was every white peak decked upon its brow with this tiara of ineffable beauty.

The impression is very general that the average quantity of snow has greatly diminished in America; but it must be remembered that very severe storms occur only at considerable intervals, and the Puritans did not always, as boys fancy, step out of the upper windows upon the snow. In 1717, the ground was covered from ten to twenty feet, indeed; but during January, 1861, the snow was six feet on a level in many parts of Maine and New Hampshire, and was probably drifted three times that depth in particular spots. The greatest storm recorded in England, I believe, is that of 1814, in which for forty-eight hours the snow fell so furiously that drifts of sixteen, twenty, and even twenty-four feet were recorded in various places. An inch an hour is thought to be the average rate of deposit, though four inches are said to have fallen during the severe storm of January 3d, 1859. When thus intensified, the "beautiful meteor of the snow" begins to give a sensation of something formidable; and when the mercury suddenly falls meanwhile, and the wind rises, there are sometimes suggestions of such terror in a snow-storm as no summer thunders can rival. The brief and singular tempest of February 7th, 1861, was a thing to be forever remembered by those who saw it, as I did, over a wide plain. The sky suddenly appeared to open and let down whole solid snow-banks at once, which were caught and torn to pieces by the ravenous winds, and the traveller was instantaneously enveloped in a whirling mass far denser than any fog; it was a tornado with snow stirred into it. Standing in the middle of the road, with houses close on every side, one could see absolutely nothing in any direction, one could hear no sound but the storm. Every landmark vanished, and it was no more possible to guess the points of the compass than in mid-ocean. It was easy to conceive of being bewildered and overwhelmed within a rod of one's own door. The tempest lasted only an hour; but if it had lasted a week, we should have had such a storm as occurred on the steppes of Kirgheez in Siberia, in 1827, destroying two hundred and eighty thousand five hundred horses, thirty thousand four hundred cattle, a million sheep, and ten thousand camels, — or as "the thirteen drifty days," in 1620, which killed nine tenths of all the sheep in the South of Scotland. On Eskdale Moor, out of twenty thousand only forty-five were left alive, and the shepherds everywhere built up huge semicircular walls of the dead creatures, to afford shelter to the living, till the gale should end. But the most remarkable narrative of a snow-storm which I have ever seen was that written by James Hogg, the Ettrick Shepherd, in record of one which took place January 24th, 1790.

James Hogg at this time belonged to a sort of literary society of young shepherds, and had set out, the day previous, to walk twenty miles over the hills to the place of meeting; but so formidable was the look of the sky that he felt anxious for his sheep, and finally turned back again. There was at that time only a slight fall of snow, in thin flakes which seemed uncertain whether to go up or down; the hills were covered with deep folds of frost-fog, and in the valleys the same fog seemed dark, dense, and as it were crushed together. An old shepherd, predicting a storm, bade him watch for a sudden opening through this fog, and expect a wind from that quarter; yet when he saw such an opening suddenly form at midnight, (having then reached his own home,) he thought it all a delusion, as the weather had grown milder and a thaw seemed setting in. He therefore went to bed, and felt no more anxiety for his sheep; yet he lay awake in spite of himself, and at two o'clock he heard the storm begin. It smote the house suddenly, like a great peal of thunder, — something utterly unlike any storm he had ever before heard. On his rising and thrusting his bare arm through a hole in the roof, it seemed precisely as if he had thrust it into a snow-bank, so densely was the air filled with falling and driving particles. He lay still for an hour, while the house rocked with the tempest, hoping it might prove only a hurricane; but as there was no abatement, he wakened his companion-shepherd, telling him "it was come on such a night or morning as never blew from the heavens." The other at once arose, and, opening the door of the shed where they slept, found a drift as high as the farm-house already heaped between them and its walls, a distance of only fourteen yards. He floundered through, Hogg soon following, and, finding all the family up, they agreed that they must reach the sheep as soon as possible, especially eight hundred ewes that were in one lot together, at the farthest end of the farm.

So, after family-prayers and breakfast, four of them stuffed their pockets with bread and cheese, sewed their plaids about them, tied down their hats, and, taking each his staff, set out on their tremendous undertaking, two hours before day.

Day dawned before they got three hundred yards from the house. They could not see each other, and kept together with the greatest difficulty. They had to make paths with their staves, rolled themselves over drifts otherwise impassable, and every three or four minutes had to hold their heads down between their knees to recover breath. They went in single file, taking the lead by turns. The master soon gave out, and was speechless and semi-conscious for more than an hour, though he afterwards recovered and held out with the rest. Two of them lost their head-gear, and Hogg himself fell over a high precipice; but they reached the flock at half past ten. They found the ewes huddled together in a dense body, under ten feet of snow, — packed so closely, that, to the amazement of the shepherds, when they had extricated the first, the whole flock walked out one after another, in a body, through the hole.

How they got them home it is almost impossible to tell. It was now noon, and they sometimes could see through the storm for twenty yards, but they had only one momentary glimpse of the hills through all that terrible day. Yet Hogg persisted in going by himself afterwards to rescue some flocks of his own, barely escaping with life from the expedition; his eyes were sealed up with the storm, and he crossed a formidable torrent, without knowing it, on a wreath of snow. Two of the others lost themselves in a deep valley, and would have perished but for being accidentally heard by a neighboring shepherd, who guided them home, where the female portion of the family had abandoned all hope of ever seeing them again.

The next day was clear, with a cold wind, and they set forth again at daybreak to seek the remainder of the flock. The face of the country was perfectly transformed: not a hill was the same, not a brook or lake could be recognized. Deep glens were filled in with snow, covering the very tops of the trees; and over a hundred acres of ground, under an average depth of six or eight feet, they were to look for four or five hundred sheep. The attempt would have been hopeless but for a dog that accompanied them: seeing their perplexity, he began snuffing about, and presently scratching in the snow at a certain point, and then looking round at his master: digging at this spot, they found a sheep beneath. And so the dog led them all day, bounding eagerly from one place to another, much faster than they could dig the creatures out, so that he sometimes had twenty or thirty holes marked beforehand. In this way, within a week, they got out every sheep on the farm except four, these last being buried under a mountain of snow fifty feet deep, on the top of which the dog had marked their places again and again. In every case the sheep proved to be alive and warm, though half suffocated; on being taken out, they usually bounded away swiftly, and then fell helplessly in a few moments, overcome by the change of atmosphere; some then died almost instantly, and others were carried home and with difficulty preserved, only about sixty being lost in all. Marvellous to tell, the country-people unanimously agreed afterwards to refer the whole terrific storm to some secret incantations of poor Hogg's literary society aforesaid; it was generally maintained that a club of young dare-devils had raised the Fiend himself among them in the likeness of a black dog, the night preceding the storm, and the young students actually did not dare to show themselves at fairs or at markets for a year afterwards.

Snow-scenes less exciting, but more wild and dreary, may be found in Alexander Henry's Travels with the Indians, in the last century. In the winter of 1776, for instance, they wandered for many hundred miles over the farthest northwestern prairies, where scarcely a white man had before trodden. The snow lay from four to six feet deep. They went on snow-shoes, drawing their stores on sleds. The mercury was sometimes —32°; no fire could keep them warm at night, and often they had no fire, being scarcely able to find wood enough to melt the snow for drink. They lay beneath buffalo-skins and the stripped bark of trees: a foot of snow sometimes fell on them before morning. The sun rose at half past nine and set at half past two. "The country was one uninterrupted plain, in many parts of which no wood, nor even the smallest shrub, was to be seen: a frozen sea, of which the little coppices were the islands. That behind which we had encamped the night before soon sank in the horizon, and the eye had nothing left save only the sky and snow." Fancy them encamped by night, seeking shelter in a scanty grove from a wild tempest of snow; then suddenly charged upon by a herd of buffaloes, thronging in from all sides of the wood to take shelter likewise, — the dogs barking, the Indians firing, and still the bewildered beasts rushing madly in, blinded by the storm, fearing the guns within less than the fury without, crashing through the trees, trampling over the tents, and falling about in the deep and dreary snow! No other writer has ever given us the full desolation of Indian winter-life. Whole families, Henry said, frequently perished together in such storms. No wonder that the aboriginal legends are full of "mighty Peboan, the Winter," and of Kabibonokka in his lodge of snow-drifts.

The interest inspired by these simple narratives suggests the reflection, that literature, which has thus far portrayed so few aspects of external Nature, has described almost nothing of winter beauty. In English books, especially, this season is simply forlorn and disagreeable, dark and dismal.

> "And foul and fierce
> All winter drives along the darkened air."

> "When dark December shrouds the transient day,
> And stormy winds are howling in their ire,
> Why com'st not thou? . . . . . O, haste to pay
> The cordial visit sullen hours require!"

> "Winter will oft at eve resume the breeze,
> Chill the pale morn, and bid his driving blasts
> Deform the day delightless."

> "Now that the fields are dank and ways are mire,
> With whom you might converse, and by the fire
> Help waste the sullen day."

But our prevalent association with winter, in the Northern United States, is with something white and dazzling and brilliant; and it is time to paint our own pictures, and cease to borrow these gloomy alien tints. One must turn eagerly every season to the few glimpses of American winter aspects: to Emerson's "Snow-Storm," every word a sculpture; to the admirable storm in "Margaret"; to Thoreau's "Winter Walk," in the "Dial"; and to Lowell's "First Snow-Flake." These are fresh and real pictures, which carry us back to the Greek Anthology, where the herds come wandering down from the wooded mountains, covered with snow, and to Homer's aged Ulysses, his wise words falling like the snows of winter.

Let me add to this scanty gallery of snow-pictures the quaint lore contained in one of the multitudinous sermons of Increase Mather, printed in 1704, entitled "A Brief Discourse concerning the Prayse due to God for His Mercy in giving Snow like Wool." One can fancy the delight of the oppressed Puritan boys in the days of the nineteenthlies, driven to the place of worship by the tithing-men, and cooped up on the pulpit and gallery stairs under charge of the constables, at hearing for once a discourse which they could understand, — snowballing spiritualized. This was not one of Emerson's terrible examples, — "the storm real, and the preacher only phenomenal"; but this setting of snow-drifts, which in our winters lends such grace to every stern rock and rugged tree, throws a charm even around the grim theology of the Mathers. Three main propositions, seven subdivisions, four applications, and four uses, but the wreaths and the gracefulness are cast about them all, — while the wonderful commonplace-books of those days, which held everything, had accumulated scraps of winter learning which cannot be spared from these less abstruse pages.

Beginning first at the foundation, the preacher must prove, "Prop. I. *That the Snow is fitly resembled to Wool.* Snow like Wool, sayes the Psalmist. And not only the Sacred Writers, but others make use of this Comparison. The Grecians of old were wont to call the Snow ERIODES HUDOR, *Wooly Water*, or wet Wool. The Latin word *Floccus* signifies both a Lock of Wool and a Flake of Snow, in that they resemble one another. The aptness of the similitude appears in three things." "1. In respect of the Whiteness thereof." "2. In respect of Softness." "3. In respect of that Warming Vertue that does attend the Snow." [Here the reasoning must not be omitted.] "Wool is warm. We say, *As warm as Wool*. Woolen-cloth has a greater warmth than other Cloathing has. The wool on Sheep keeps them warm in the Winter season. So when the back of the Ground is covered with Snow, it keeps it warm. Some mention it as one of the wonders of the Snow, that tho' it is itself cold, yet it makes the Earth warm. But Naturalists observe that there is a saline spirit in it, which is hot, by means whereof Plants under the Snow are kept from freezing. Ice under the Snow is sooner melted and broken than other Ice. In some Northern Climates, the wild barbarous People use to cover themselves over with it to keep them warm. When the sharp Air has begun to freeze a man's Limbs, Snow will bring heat into them again. If persons Eat much Snow, or drink immoderately of Snow-water, it will burn their Bowels and make them black. So that it has a warming vertue in it, and is therefore fitly compared to Wool."

Snow has many merits. "In *Lapland*, where there is little or no light of the sun in the depth of Winter, there are great Snows continually on the ground, and by the Light of that they are able to Travel from one place to another. . . . . . At this day in some hot Countreys, they have their Snow-cellars, where it is kept in Summer, and if moderately used, is known to be both refreshing and healthful. There are also Medicinal Vertues in the snow. A late Learned Physician has found that a *Salt* extracted out of snow is a sovereign Remedy against both putrid and pestilential Feavors. Therefore Men should Praise God, who giveth Snow like Wool." But there is an account against the snow, also. "Not only the disease called *Bulimia*, but others more fatal have come out of the Snow. *Geographers* give us to understand that in some Countries Vapours from the Snow have killed multitudes in less than a Quarter of an Hour. Sometimes both Men and Beasts have been destroyed thereby. Writers speak of no less than Forty Thousand men killed by a great Snow in one Day."

It gives a touching sense of human sympathy, to find that we may look at Orion and the Pleiades through the grave eyes of a Puritan divine. "The *Seven Stars* are the Summer Constellation: they bring on the spring and summer; and *Orion* is a Winter Constellation, which is attended with snow and cold, as at this Day. . . . . . Moreover, Late *Philosophers* by the help of the *Microscope* have observed the wonderful Wisdom of God in the Figure of the Snow; each flake is usually of a *Stellate* Form, and of six Angles of exact equal length from the Center. It is *like a little Star*. A great man speaks of it with admiration, that in a Body so familiar as the Snow is, no Philosopher should for many Ages take notice of a thing so obvious as the Figure of it. The learned *Kepler*, who lived in this last Age, is acknowledged to be the first that acquainted the world with the Sexangular Figure of the Snow."

Then come the devout applications. "There is not a Flake of Snow that falls on the Ground without the hand of God, Mat. 10. 29. 30. Not a Sparrow falls to the Ground, without the Will of your Heavenly Father, all the Hairs of your head are numbred. So the Great God has numbred all the Flakes of Snow that covers the Earth. Altho' no man can number them, that God that tells the number of the Stars has numbred them all. . . . . We often see it, when the Ground is bare, if God speaks the word, the Earth is covered with snow in a few Minutes' time. Here is the power of the Great God. If all the Princes and Great Ones of the Earth should send their Commands to the Clouds, not a Flake of snow would come from thence."

Then follow the "uses," at last, — the little boys in the congregation having grown uneasy long since, at hearing so much theorizing about snow-drifts, with so little opportunity of personal practice. "Use I. If we should Praise God for His giving Snow, surely then we ought to Praise Him for Spiritual Blessings much more." "Use II. We should Humble our selves under the Hand of God, when Snow in the season of it is witheld from us." "Use III. Hence all Atheists will be left Eternally Inexcusable." "Use IV. We should hence Learn to make a Spiritual Improvement of the Snow." And then with a closing volley of every text which figures under the head of "Snow" in the Concordance, the discourse comes to an end; and every liberated urchin goes home with his head full of devout fancies of building a snow-fort, after sunset, from which to propel consecrated missiles against imaginary or traditional Pequots.

And the patient reader, too long snow-bound, must be liberated also. After the winters of deepest drifts the spring often comes most suddenly; there is little frost in the ground, and the liberated waters, free without the expected freshet, are filtered into the earth, or climb on ladders of sunbeams to the sky. The beautiful crystals all melt away, and the places where they lay are silently made ready to be submerged in new drifts of summer ver ure. These also will be transmuted in their turn, and so the eternal cycle of the season glides along.

Near my house there is a garden, beneath whose stately

sycamores a fountain plays. Three sculptured girls lift forever upward a chalice which distils unceasingly a fine and plashing rain; in summer the spray holds the maidens in a glittering veil, but winter takes the radiant drops and slowly builds them up into a shroud of ice which creeps gradually about the three slight figures: the feet vanish, the waist is encircled, the head is covered, the piteous uplifted arms disappear, as if each were a Vestal Virgin entombed alive for her transgression. They vanishing entirely, the fountain yet plays on unseen; all winter the pile of ice grows larger, glittering organ-pipes of congelation add themselves outside, and by February a great glacier is formed, at whose buried centre stand immovably the patient girls. Spring comes at last, the fated prince, to free with glittering spear these enchanted beauties; the waning glacier, slowly receding, lies conquered before their liberated feet; and still the fountain plays. Who can despair before the iciest human life, when its unconscious symbols are so beautiful?

Cambridge: Stereotyped and Printed by Welch, Bigelow, & Co.

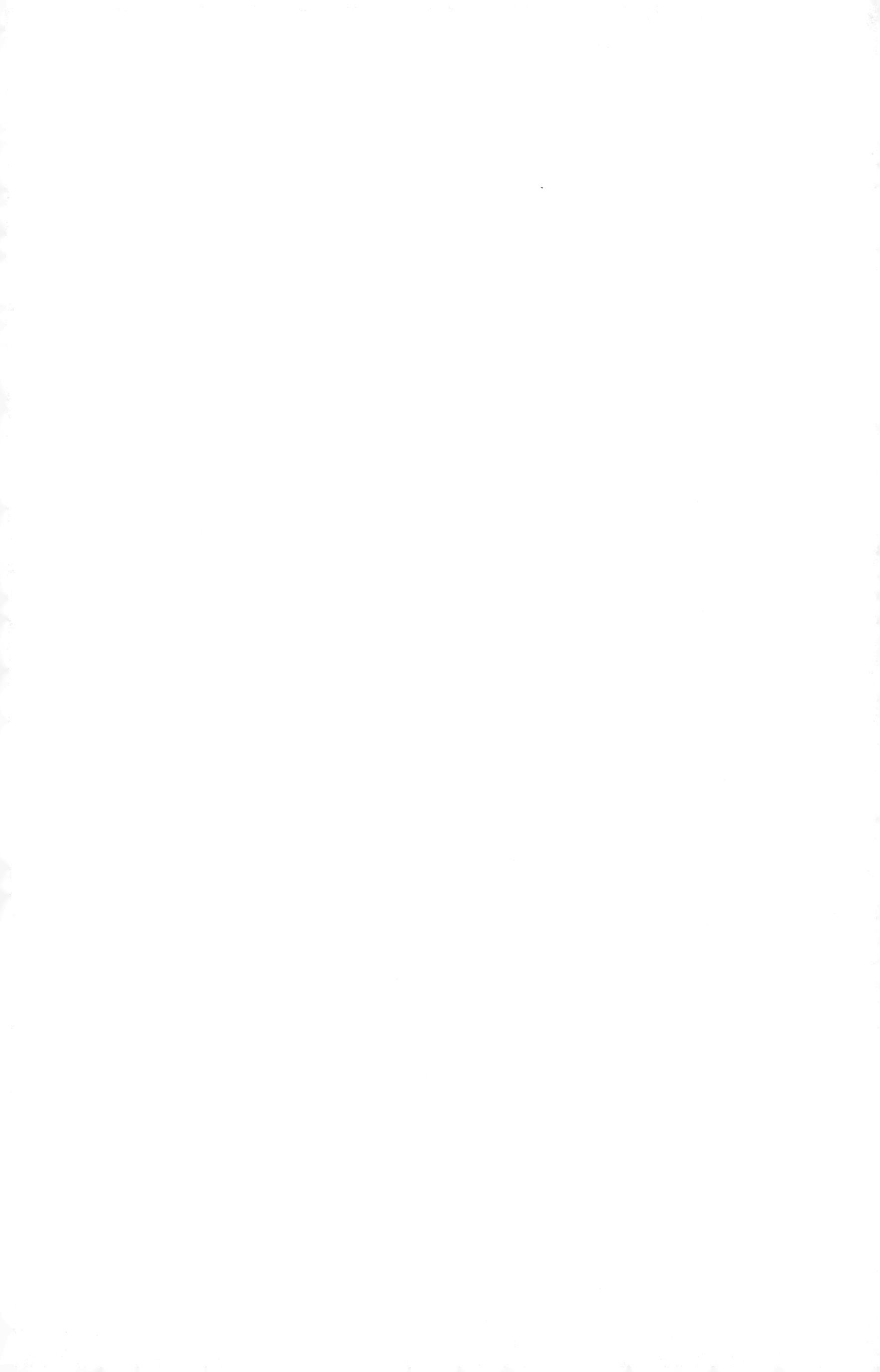

www.ingramcontent.com/pod-product-compliance
Lightning Source LLC
LaVergne TN
LVHW010131110826
845151LV00002B/330

* 9 7 8 1 4 2 5 5 3 9 8 6 3 *